CRITICAL THINKING IN MEDICAL-SURGICAL SETTINGS: A Case Study Approach

Second Edition

by

Maryl L. Winningham, APRN, PhD, FACSM
Executive Director and Senior Research Fellow
Institute for the Advancement of Health Care Engineering
Salt Lake City, Utah

and

Barbara A. Preusser, PhD, FNPc
Family Nurse Practitioner
Veteran's Administration Medical Center
Salt Lake City, Utah

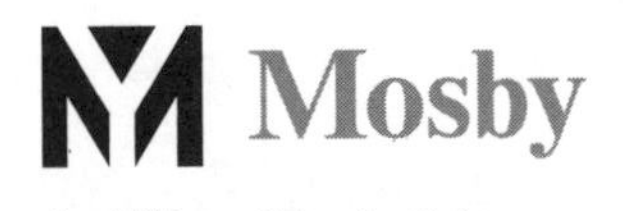

An Affiliate of Elsevier Science

St. Louis London Philadelphia Sydney Toronto

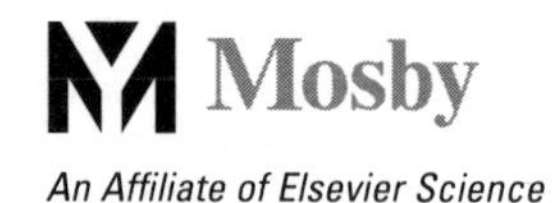

An Affiliate of Elsevier Science

Vice President, Nursing Editorial Director: Sally Schrefer
Senior Editor: Michael S. Ledbetter
Senior Developmental Editor: Laurie Muench
Project Manager: Gayle May Morris
Cover Designer: Julia Ramirez

SECOND EDITION

NOTICE
Pharmacology is an ever-changing field. Standard safety precautions must be followed, but as new research and clinical experience broaden our knowledge, changes in treatment and drug therapy may become necessary or appropriate. Readers are advised to check the most current product information provided by the manufacturer of each drug to be administered to verify the recommended dose, the method and duration of administration, and contraindications. It is the responsibility of the appropriately licensed health care provider, relying on experience and knowledge of the patient, to determine dosages and the best treatment for each individual patient. Neither the publisher nor the editor assumes any liability for any injury and/or damage to persons or property arising from this publication.

Mosby, Inc.
An Affiliate of Elsevier Science
11830 Westline Industrial Drive
St. Louis, Missouri 63146

Printed in the United States of America

International Standard Book Number: 0-323-01154-3

03 04 WB/EB 9 8 7 6 5 4

Clinical Consultants

Clinical Nursing Practice
Kathy Evans, BSN
Staff Nurse and Diabetes Educator
University of Utah Health Sciences Center
Salt Lake City, Utah

Pharmacy
Karen Gunning, PharmD
Director, Clinical Pharmacy
University of Utah College of Pharmacy
Salt Lake City, Utah

Laboratory Science
Linda Olinger, BS, BSMT, ASCP
Laboratory Science Consultant
Akron, Ohio

Nutrition
Linda J. Winningham, MS, RD
Nutritional Consultant
Ray, Michigan

Clinical Advisors

K. Louise Long, RN
LDS Hospital
Salt Lake City, Utah

Jeanine Smith, RN
LDS Hospital
Salt Lake City, Utah

Reviewer

Susan J. W. Hsia, PhD, RN, MS, MN
Associate Professor, School of Nursing
Washburn University
Topeka, Kansas

Dedication

To Galileo Galilei, pioneer in the process

of scientific "Thought Experiment"

and martyr to scientific freedom of inquiry and thought;

to Florence Nightingale, who taught us

that careful observation is the basis for modern nursing;

and to all those who dare to lead the way into the future

with new ideas while others are still saying,

"We've never done it that way before."

M.L.W. and B.A.P

Acknowledgments

We would like to thank:

Our patients, who let us learn nursing by practicing on them.

Those nurses we saw in action and told ourselves, "Now *that's* a great nurse!"

The teachers who encouraged us to follow our convictions.

And to those who have bequeathed to us a nursing heritage of integrity, excellence, courage, and service.

To them we humbly acknowledge our gratitude and indebtedness.

This book would never have become a reality if not for the forbearance and help of the following individuals:

Michael Ledbetter, Senior Editor, who made this book a reality and has shared his patience, encouragement, and compassion;

Laurie Muench, Senior Developmental Editor, who tried to keep us on the straight and narrow, patiently listened to us complain, coordinated the review process, and edited this work. Laurie, thank you for the great person you are;

Laurie Selkirk, Senior Editorial Assistant, for her support.

And our consultants, for the creative work they shared with us and for their sharp eyes that picked up on errors. We thank you for your unflagging support.

We would like to offer a special tribute to the people who said, "It can't be done," "It'll never work," and "We've never done it that way," and thereby challenged us to prove them wrong.

M.L.W.

B.A.P.

Table of Contents

Student Introduction

This is a *process* manual, not a workbook. It is designed to help you learn a whole new way of thinking: thinking like a good nurse. No one can *make* you learn. Learning happens. It is a *process* in which exposure to certain information and experiences comes together to create something new in your mind. Motivation, the stimulus to learning, can be negative or positive. In negative situations, you learn because you are threatened by fear. Examples include bad grades (fear of failure) and looking stupid (fear of humiliation). Positive motivation to learn involves feeling good about yourself or seeing a benefit to learning. In other words, you *want* to learn. Examples of this include wanting to look like you know what you are doing, wanting to feel successful, and being challenged by something that interests you.

Human beings can be motivated simply by interest. There is some built-in mechanism that makes our minds want to grow and learn. One of the best ways to positively motivate is through *relevance*. Relevance involves learning because you are interested in something or because you see it as useful to you. All the cases in this book are based on real-life clinical experiences. Within a few years, people's lives will be in your hands. The knowledge you possess and the decisions you make will have a significant impact. We hope that by using true, clinically based examples, you experience motivation through relevance. Like a Sherlock Holmes story, each case represents a mystery with many clues. It will be up to you to put those clues together, ask the right questions, identify the right resources, draw the right conclusions, and put it all together to solve your case. Faculty members, facilitators, or teachers are called "instructors" in this book. Instructors are there to help you find the critical information, collect your clues, and figure out how to put them together. Solving the case will mean doing what is best for the person(s) in your case study.

Throughout this book, we refer to persons in the cases as "patients." We use the word "patient" because there are certain legal obligations that nurses are held to by law and those relationships are defined as nurse-patient relationships. Some instructors may refer to them as "clients" or by some other term. Use the term your instructor prefers. The important thing is—no matter what we call them—they are human beings who deserve the best care we can provide.

As we wrote this book, we thought of you. We did our best to help you work through the difficult transition from words to action, from lecture and textbook to the clinical setting. We were both students for many years, and we understand how boring or frustrating the learning experience can seem. We also know how easy it is to become discouraged. Give yourself a break. The learning process inside the brain is a fascinating thing: at the very time you think you are making the least progress, you may be unconsciously preparing yourself to develop insight into a whole new way of thinking.

Maryl L. Winningham, APRN, PhD, FACSM
and
Barbara A. Preusser, PhD, FNPc
Salt Lake City, Utah, 2000

Critical Thinking and Case Studies: Getting Started

Introduction

This chapter starts with a discussion of what critical thinking is and what case studies are. This is followed by a section with tips about how to solve case studies. You will discover that solving a case study is much like working a puzzle or unraveling a mystery. Also included are two brief stories about the best and worst nurses we (the authors) have ever met. The first story shows you that memorization and grades alone do not make a good nurse. The second story illustrates that it takes time and self-confidence to become a good nurse—and that you need to be patient with yourself. Following the stories are two case studies that we will walk you through, step by step, to give you an idea of how all this fits together. In each case, you will learn a little more about the process of discovering clues, learning the art of self-correction, and the importance of being able to take what you have learned in this course (as well as others) and apply it to the practice of thinking through cases.

In the Appendices we have provided helpful materials for you. Take a look at them now. In Appendix A, a section called **Pointers for Students** consists of tips contributed by people who helped us write this book. By reading a few of these at a time and practicing applying them, you should start to look and feel like a good clinician. Appendix B includes a form called **Case Study Worksheet**. Do not write on the sheet in the Appendix. If you legally purchased this book, you have permission to make as many photocopies of this form as you need. On the form you will notice areas marked "___ Preparation" and "___ Self-Correction"; this allows the form to serve double-duty. You can use it to prepare your cases, learning to gather the information critical to solving them. In this case, place a check mark in the blank next to "**Preparation**." At first you will want to staple this to the back of your case study when you turn it in to your instructor. Finding the right information—gathering your clues—is the most important first step to carry out. By collecting your **Worksheet** when you first prepare your cases, your instructor has a chance to see whether you are having any problems gathering the information you need. Later, if you have trouble with certain questions, you can fill out another copy of the form—this time marked as "✓ **Self Correction**." This step is especially important when your instructor notices that your information base may be responsible for some of the problems you are having.

Strategies for Action

There are two overriding purposes to the way these cases are arranged—because learning critical thinking goes two ways. You see, instructors need feedback to analyze (think through) how you are doing. The first purpose is to help you learn the process of thinking. The second purpose is to give your instructor clues about where you may be having problems. Together, this helps you become a team, looking for strategies to help you learn to function in this whole new language and new culture—the culture of health care and nursing. Team work is essential: you must know you are never alone in this.

What Is Critical Thinking and What Are Case Studies?

Learning is usually easier when you see a reason for it. All the cases in this book are based on real-life clinical situations. As you work through these cases, we hope you will begin to understand how to take what you are learning from your books and in the classroom and apply it to patient care settings. In addition, we hope it will help you gain insight into how experienced nurses think.

We know that "A" students do not always make the best nurses. On the other hand, the "B" or "C" student may become an excellent nurse. Why? Memorization and regurgitation of "book learning" is not enough to make you a good nurse. The key is application. Learning to "think on your feet" means being able to apply quickly what you know in practical, everyday situations. Learners are drawn to information they believe is relevant and interesting; they are bored when they think certain information is irrelevant. Relevance can be experienced through realistic simulations. Furthermore, critical thinking is an interactive process. This process occurs when you:

1. Encounter challenges (clinical exposure to problems);

2. Need to find information to solve those problems (gather data);
3. Attempt to solve a problem (need to react in a clinical situation);
4. Obtain feedback regarding the usefulness of that information (always consider the possibility of insufficient or incorrect data) and whether that information can be applied in a useful way (decide on a plan);
5. Revise your strategy toward obtaining more data or considering different ways of applying it to the problem (rethink your game plan); and
6. Are rewarded by the satisfaction of new levels of understanding and positive outcomes (you notice you are starting to catch on more quickly and function more smoothly).

To help you learn, the instructor (facilitator, teacher, faculty member) can help by providing an environment with opportunities for problem solving and self-correction.

What Is Critical Thinking?

First, let us talk about what critical thinking is *not*. It is not criticizing. Rather, it is an analytical process that can help you think through a problem in an organized and efficient manner. Half a century ago, two writers suggested there were six steps involved in critical thinking (Dressel and Mayhew, 1954). Thinking about these steps may help you when you work through the questions in your cases. In the beginning, it may help for you to write everything down, step by step, as you learn the process of discovery. Here are the six steps with an explanation of what they mean.

1. **Define the problem by asking the right questions:** Exactly what is it you need to know? What is the question asking? Einstein once said that asking the right question was sometimes more important than having the right answer.
2. **Select the information or data necessary to solve the problem or answer the question:** First, you have to ask whether all the necessary data or information is there. If not, how and where can you get additional information? What other resources are available? This is one of the most difficult steps. In real clinical experiences, you rarely have all the information, so you have to learn where you can get necessary data. For instance, patient and family interviews, patient nursing charts, patient medical charts, laboratory data on the computer, your observations, and your own physical assessment can help you identify important clues. Of course, information can rapidly become outdated. To make sure you are accessing the most current and accurate information, you will occasionally need to use a computer and the Internet to answer a question.
3. **Recognize stated and unstated assumptions; that is, what do you think is or is not true?** Assumptions can be dangerous. The following two statements—although they may sound obvious at first—can help you avoid relying on assumptions:
   a. *"You never find an answer you don't think of."* Sometimes answers or solutions seem obvious. To jump on an answer or solution too quickly may lead you astray. Just because something seems obvious doesn't mean it is correct. Search your mind to see whether there are other possible answers to the question or solutions to the problem. You may miss the right answer because you assume it is something else. In short, *don't get hung up on the obvious* and *when something looks obvious, try to find another reason.*
   b. *"Don't discard a potential answer too quickly."* You may need to consider several possible answers or solutions. What if you decide something can't possibly be true? You throw it away in your mind. But what if you actually throw away the right solution? Consider all clues carefully and *don't dismiss a possibility too quickly.*
4. **Formulate and select relevant and/or promising hypotheses:** Think of these as hunches. Try to think of as many possibilities as you can. Consider the "pros" and "cons" of each. If you find yourself having trouble recognizing the pros and cons, take a sheet of paper, draw a line straight down the middle of the page, and put "Con" (against the argument) at the top of the left column and "Pro" (supportive of the argument) at the top of the right one. Setting up this simple chart can sometimes "jump start" the process of weighing your options.
5. **Draw valid conclusions:** Consider all data; then determine what is relevant and what makes the most sense. Only then should you draw your conclusions.

6. **Consider the soundness of your decisions:** Rethink your conclusions and decisions in light of the whole case. What is the best answer/solution? What could go wrong? This requires considering many different angles. Be willing to revise the conclusions you made in step 5 if new information or clues crop up. In today's health care settings, decision making often requires balancing the well-being and needs of the patient with financial limitations imposed by the reimbursement system (this includes Medicare, Medicaid, and insurance companies). In making decisions, you need to take all the relevant issues into account. Remember, you may be asked to explain why you rejected other options.

It may look as if this kind of thinking comes naturally to instructors or experienced nurses. You may also think this sounds impossible for you, especially if you are just starting your program. You can be certain that even experienced professionals were once where you are now. (Sometimes they seem to forget that!) The rapid and sound decision making that is essential to good nursing requires years of practice. The practice of good clinical thinking leads to good thinking in clinical practice. This book will help you practice the important steps in making sound, clinical judgments again and again, until the process starts to come naturally. In reality, "naturally" is the result of a lot good thinking—it does not just "happen" accidentally. To pull together the many kinds of information necessary for these cases, you will need to draw on everything you have learned in your prerequisite courses and what you are learning in your nursing courses. This process will bring a whole new level of relevance to what you are learning.

The practice of good clinical thinking leads to good thinking in clinical practice.

The questions or problems related to cases in this book fall into one of the following five categories, each building on the last. That is, each category requires a more sophisticated level of thinking than the previous. Sometimes different types of questions or problems will be mixed together in the same case. If you are confused about a question, try breaking it down step by step.

Knowledge—This represents information, data, or facts and deals with questions like Who? What? When? Where? and How much?

Comprehension—This involves understanding the importance, significance, or meaning of specific information or facts.

Application—This involves understanding the information or facts and implementing or using them. Application also involves figuring out what—of all the information in a given setting—is important and appropriate to the problem and applying that information to a plan of action. Each setting contains a lot of information; some of it is not relevant. In some settings, certain information may even lead us to false conclusions.

Analysis—This involves criticism and evaluation and requires taking a situation or problem apart to figure out what is going on (or going wrong). Analysis involves knowledge, understanding the meaning or significance of that knowledge, and recognizing how it can best be applied. It also involves evaluating ("figuring out") what is wrong or anticipating what can go wrong. In finding out what is wrong, you will encounter one or more assumptions that may lead to false conclusions or something that you don't understand.

Synthesis—This is a more advanced kind of thinking that requires combining, arranging, incorporating, integrating, or coordinating what you know to arrive at a specific result. Synthesis is a creative process that involves pulling everything together. This type of thinking is characteristic of advanced clinicians. In a deeper sense, although the questions in these cases are not synthesis-type questions, your brain is constantly in "synthesis mode." Indeed, that's why case studies help develop your clinical thinking skills—they help you learn to synthesize new brain structures in a way that memorization cannot.

Most of the questions in this book will involve the first four types of thinking. In general, any given situation requires:

1. Knowing certain facts;
2. Understanding what they mean;
3. Being able to individualize and apply them in your setting;
4. Figuring out what is going on (taking it apart in your mind); and
5. Reconsidering the facts, what they mean, and how to apply them.

What Are Case Studies?

Case studies capture key elements in a clinical situation. They are like snapshots of a scenario during a specific period in time. You are asked to evaluate that snapshot and answer certain questions. Facts or data are given to you in the case; however, not all the necessary information is provided. This is where the mystery begins. Some of the information comes from your prior educational experiences (e.g., lectures, books, clinical assignments), some comes directly from the case ("snapshot"), some you will research in texts and references, and some you will develop from the information provided (the problem-solving part). In other words, some clues are provided in the case, some are things you already know, and some will have to be discovered by using resources and asking yourself the right questions.

The questions will walk you through a sequence of problems or activities, so "the plot thickens" as you work through the case. This will guide you in a process of self-discovery. Books, lectures, and other resources are important because they provide you with necessary background information. In each case, information about the patient provides you with more specific clues. The most important part, though, is how you bring it all together to make it "happen" in your mind. Using case studies or case-based reasoning has proved to be an effective learning method in many professional programs, including business, law, engineering, and medicine.

The Secret of "Success Imaging"

One of the most powerful tools used by coaches and sports psychologists in training athletes is "success imaging." This method becomes particularly important when athletes feel attacked by their own self-doubt and fear of failure. (Does that sound familiar?) Success imaging helps athletes improve their self-confidence and performance. In this process, athletes are taught to make "mind movies" in which they picture themselves successfully going through the process of their sport. Successful athletes spend about 90% of their practice time working on drills (basic skills). They also know their equipment. In success imaging, they picture themselves making "sweet spot" moves, perfecting their skills in their mind before they ever pick up a racket, a football, or a bat.

You share a lot in common with professional athletes, who work in high-stress situations where everything depends on their performance. In addition to high stress, you must deal with many distractions that make it difficult to concentrate. Clinical situations involve a great deal of commotion. Sometimes it is difficult to figure out what is happening. Obviously, you cannot know everything at once. The learning process is stressful in situations like this because patient care is a heavy responsibility. Currently, your work is supervised by faculty and by nurses. They are your coaches. They encourage you to polish your basic skills and acquire the knowledge you will need to grow professionally. They know that errors in judgment or lack of knowledge in a clinical setting can result in harm to a patient and to your career. Soon you will be the nurse, and the decision-making responsibility with fall upon you. As a professional, you will be teaching others. You will come to know the pride of seeing your former assistants and students become polished nurses.

To use success imaging in case studies, work through the cases as outlined in the following discussion. Then go back, read through each case, and review your answers. Does your answer make sense? Close your eyes and picture what you have just read in your mind, step by step, as if the patient were a real person in front of you, and you were a nurse in that setting. Picture yourself observing the situation, making your assessment, performing—step by step—the necessary skills, looking at the labels on drug bottles, drawing up doses, interacting with the patient and the family, and so on.

Think through what is happening, and why, in slow motion. Does it flow? If not, perhaps something is missing or inaccurate. This is a chance to go back and engage in self-correction, examining your answers in your mind for flaws or to see whether something has been ignored or left out. "Image" through the case again, as if you were playing back a video tape for an "instant replay" in your mind.

Finally, the best test comes when you mentally "success image" yourself teaching and demonstrating that case to someone else. That means you have managed to creatively integrate all kinds of information in finding solutions. Congratulate yourself!

The Principle of "Specificity of Training"

Another important principle used by coaches and trainers is called "specificity of training." The meaning is simple: If you want to become a better swimmer, practice swimming. Your swimming is not improved by chewing gum or playing golf. You learn as much as you can about swimming. You work on perfecting your stroke. You practice the basic skills again and again, gradually increasing in speed and becoming more efficient and accurate. Quite simply, you learn to do something well when you practice it again and again. You build your confidence by perfecting your basic skills, day by day and step by step.

As in athletics, the key to becoming a better nurse is to practice thinking like a good nurse. Case studies let you practice clinically relevant thought processes in a less stressful environment without the risk—or stress—of embarrassing yourself or hurting someone else. Nursing is a complex and challenging profession. People learn best when they can experiment, take chances, and even be allowed to make mistakes. Furthermore, they are able to apply what they have learned when they can use their building blocks of knowledge. Experience and practice are the mortar. In case studies, you learn by studying the questions and searching for answers. Then, you put them together by applying them to the decisions you make.

You often learn more, and faster, when you have the freedom to make mistakes and then have the chance to correct yourself. Because correction takes longer, you develop your own positive reinforcement for being more careful and accurate the next time. This book is designed to allow you to experiment with finding answers. More important, it helps you learn a whole new process of thinking—thinking like a good nurse. If you miss the point the first time, it will help you learn how to correct yourself and find your own solutions. One sign of a good clinician is the ability to self-correct and self-teach. Think of it as a puzzle, a mystery, or a game. Case studies allow you to learn creative ways of problem solving. You pick up little clues all over the place—the ability to make sense of many little clues is the sign of a good detective. Welcome to the mystery, Sherlock!

What Is Self-Correction?

Figuring out where you went wrong and how to correct it is a much more self-reinforcing learning technique than just having someone tell you what you did wrong. On the other hand, you often need some guidance to point you in the right direction. Self-correction is a process whereby you review your response to a problem to figure out how you can improve. It is a process that is essential to applying critical thinking in nursing. In self-correction, you go back to the beginning of the problem and ask:

1. Do I have all the necessary information? Am I missing something? Is my information inaccurate, outdated, or incomplete?
2. Do I understand what the problem means? Perhaps there are several meanings, or I don't understand the problem or the meaning of data.
3. Am I matching the correct information with the specific problem in this particular setting? This requires individualizing the information. For example, one of the best ways to do this with medications is to ask whether the disease(s) and the drugs match.
4. Do I really understand the whole picture? What is missing? What is not necessary or incorrect?

Beside each question or problem statement in this book, there is a set of check boxes that are part of a feedback coding system. This is to help your instructor communicate with you to let you know whether you need to self-correct your response to a problem and guide you about what kind of correction should be made. This system will be explained further in association with Sample Case Study 2 in this chapter.

So Who Cares About Critical Thinking?

There is an urgent need for nurses with well-practiced critical thinking skills. New graduates are often expected to make decisions and take actions of an increasingly sophisticated nature. Frequently, these nurses encounter problems they never saw or heard about during their student clinical experiences. The need to consider the complexity of a problem in decision making, along with a wide variety of variables (e.g., social, emotional, physical, financial, spiritual), is unprecedented. Furthermore, these decisions must be made in clinical settings with little guidance and limited resources. In this chapter, you will read several case study samples. We will walk through them with you, step by step, so that you can experience what it is like to creatively work through case studies. Do not be discouraged if you don't seem to catch on immediately. Success at solving case studies is cumulative; that is, you improve with each case. In addition, *each person learns in a different way and at a different pace*. Sometimes those who appear to be catching on more slowly make the best nurses—it just takes them more time to learn in their own special way. Have respect for your unique abilities, and resist the temptation to compare your progress with others.

The Problem with Grades

It is difficult to "grade" case studies. At first, students often prefer the security of objective tests and quizzes, such as multiple choice and true-false tests. Unfortunately, as you know, real life does not lend itself to the simplicity of these methods. Real-life situations are complex, ambiguous, constantly changing, and confusing, including problems to which there are no "right" answers. More commonly, we are stuck with having to do the best we can with what we have. Developing an understanding of how to deal with ambiguity (think of this as "mental fuzziness") is a sign of professional maturity. The people who frequently find case studies the most frustrating are those accustomed to making top grades and getting everything right. The following two stories should help you understand this a little better.

The Worst and Best Nurses We Have Known

To help you understand that being a good nurse is not just "jumping through the hoops," memorizing, and getting good grades, we are going to share an example of the worst and best nurses we have ever known. The nurses in these examples are real, but their names have been changed to protect the guilty. In reading about these two examples, we hope you are encouraged to "chill out," let yourself grow as a person, and enjoy these two true stories. You also may learn a few useful things in the process.

The Smartest Nursing Student I Ever Knew

Of the thousands of nursing students I have worked with over the years, Sylvia, one of my classmates, was the smartest one I ever met. Sylvia had a photographic memory and was very fond of informing each of her classmates the exact location (page and paragraph) of each answer to every test question. The instructors soon learned to avoid Sylvia—she would dog them day and night if they dared to deduct one-tenth of a point from her papers or tests for any reason. She would demand they change her grade. After all, she was perfect in every way. In short, Sylvia was someone everyone loved to hate.

After graduation, I obtained a position on a medical floor for terminally ill patients. I had no idea that I was about to work on the same floor as Sylvia. Every day she entertained me with her insufferable story of how the people who scored her State Board exam must have miscoded the answers because she had not gotten a perfect score. To make matters worse, my car broke down and I had to ride to and from work with Sylvia, listening to more of her daily rendition of *"How Great I Am."* I experienced alternating violent suicidal and homicidal feelings.

One day, Sylvia stopped me in the hall and asked me to help her clean up a patient. I told her I had to finish something but I would be there in five minutes. As I walked into the room, Sylvia looked at her watch, tapped her foot, and shot me a look that said, "You said you would be here in five minutes and that was 45 seconds ago." I took one look at her patient and the three little elderly women who were doting over him and whispered, "Sylvia, your patient is dead!"

"What do you mean my patient's . . ." she started whining as I firmly cupped my hand over her mouth.

I swept past Sylvia and asked the three women to please collect their purses and step outside until we got him cleaned up. I told them they didn't have to go far because we were going to ask them to come right back. I closed the door behind the last woman and whispered in an irritated voice, "Sylvia, I can't believe you! Your patient is dead as a door nail!"

"How can you tell?" Sylvia asked, in the same whiny voice.

"Well, alive people usually aren't that shade of gray and besides, your patient is not breathing! Alive people usually breathe," I informed her.

I attempted to turn the patient so that Sylvia could clean him. He was so dead rigor mortis had already set in. I explained that when patients died, the rectal sphincter dilates and the contents of the rectum evacuate. To this day, I wonder how she had obtained such convincing vital signs for the previous few hours on a dead person.

Life became a lot more tolerable after that. Every time Sylvia starting telling me how smart she was, I would cut her short with "Hey, Sylvia, this is me you're talking to. Remember the dead guy?"

Sylvia was the smartest student I ever knew, but she was a miserable failure as a nurse. She could memorize books and quote facts, but she couldn't make the transition to practice. This book is designed to help you make that transition, to help you practice applying what you are learning, and to help you learn to think and act like a good nurse.

Barbara A. Preusser, Ph.D., FNPc

The Greatest Nurse I Ever Knew

I have known many great, as well as some not-so-great, nurses in my lifetime. Of the good ones, there is one I put at the top of my list. I'll call her Mary Ann. Mary Ann grew up smack dab in the middle of a large, very average American family in a very average American neighborhood. Her father drove a truck, and her mother suffered from mental illness, a burden that affected the entire family. All the way through school, she was a slightly-above-average student, not outstanding in anything. She graduated from a diploma nursing program. She was kind of quiet. She never impressed anyone as being especially gifted or brilliant.

When did she become such a good nurse? I don't know. I do know she always seemed to be a decent, kind, honest person. If I could tell you one thing about her that stood out, I would tell you she was a great listener—and she was a very patient person. Even when everyone was running around like crazy, she seemed to have a calm about her. When did she get so smart? She never made a big deal about it, but somehow she always seemed to know to do the right thing at the right time. I don't think she was what anyone would call beautiful, but I don't think any of the patients even thought about that. She was beautiful to them because she radiated a peaceful confidence that put their fears to rest. They felt safe around her. She was never a manager or administrator, never an elected leader. I think most of the people she worked with were too busy and self-absorbed to realize how good she was. If anything, some of them seemed to find her calm irritating and her quiet competence threatening.

There was a time one of her patients was dying. Nobody wanted to talk about it. The family didn't want to talk about it, and they told the attending physician not to tell him he was dying. None of the nurses talked with him about it. And the patient just got sicker and sicker and more and more scared. One day, he was Mary Ann's patient. She watched him all day, but there was so much going on, with a heavy patient load, that there was little time to talk with him. At the end of the shift, she finished her charting and clocked out. Then, she went into his room and sat on a chair by his bed. "I know you need to talk," she told him quietly, "and I know it's hard." She paused, then added, "When you're ready, I'll be here." An hour went by. And another. They were undisturbed. Nobody came to his room. Nobody wanted to. The long shadow of night crept across the room. She sat, quietly waiting. At last, he took a deep breath and spoke. He talked about living. He talked about his fear. He talked about dying. He talked, and talked, and talked. And finally, he stopped talking and took a deep breath. He closed his eyes. "Thank you," he said quietly. Then he fell into the first restful sleep in many days. Only then did Mary Ann get up and leave. Her job was done.

Mary Ann has never gotten any medals, any awards, any honors. Only a few years ago she finally went back and got her master's degree in nursing. I doubt whether the graduate faculty was particularly impressed. I'm even more certain she didn't care whether they were impressed or not. It's not the sort of thing she would value. But when people talk about the characteristics of a good nurse, she is the first person who comes to my mind. Her friendship is one of the finest treasures I have. And although I know each of us has her or his own gifts and abilities and we shouldn't compare ourselves with someone else, I can't help wishing I was a little more like Mary Ann.

Maryl L. Winningham, APRN, Ph.D., FACSM

"Real Intelligence"

Perhaps one of the best ways to summarize the previous stories is with this quote:

"Real intelligence is a creative use of knowledge, not merely an accumulation of facts."

Kenneth Winebrenner

That is exactly what Winnie the Pooh (described as "a bear of very little brain") tried to explain to his friend, Piglet:

"Rabbit's clever," said Pooh thoughtfully.

"Yes," said Piglet, "Rabbit's clever."

"And he has Brains."

"Yes," said Piglet, "Rabbit has Brains."

There was a long silence.

"I suppose," said Pooh, "that's why he never understands anything."

A. A. Milne

Little Steps

The rest of this chapter will take you through two case studies, step by step. Each case study will start with a scene and some basic information. Before you start a case, have your reference books ready so that you don't have to interrupt your concentration.

When you study, there are some books you will want to keep handy: a medical dictionary, your anatomy and physiology book, your microbiology book, your pharmacology book, your nutrition book, your nursing skills book, your assessment book, your drug manual, your laboratory and diagnostic tests book, your medical-surgical textbook, and any other references your instructor may recommend. Do not sell your books at the end of each semester or quarter; you will need them to prepare your case studies, and you will study from them when you prepare for your NCLEX ("state board" exam).

The question of what is the best for your patient is difficult to answer. The practice of health care is always changing. Even textbooks can't keep up with many of the changes. To help you prepare for your future responsibilities as a nurse, we have tried to incorporate the most recent information into the case studies. However, since nurses often have to look up the most recent information on computers, in some cases you will want to use a computer with Internet access to find the most current information available.

Don't be afraid to look things up. Standards frequently change. People who think they're too smart to look something up are dangerous. The product inserts of many medications, which contain the most recent information approved by the United States Food and Drug Administration (U.S.F.D.A. or F.D.A.), can change. Many countries have their own equivalent regulatory organizations. Keep in mind that the drug names and information contained in this book may vary depending on where you are. That is a good reason why you should become familiar with the generic names of drugs. Rather than throwing product inserts away, keep them to study later.

The "How To" of Case Studies

When you begin each case, read through the whole story once, from start to finish, to get a general idea what it is about. Then go back and underline the words you don't understand. Get out your **Case Study Worksheet** and mark "**✓ Preparation**." This is your "cheat sheet." For your convenience, a copy of this form is provided at the end of both cases in this chapter. Go through the practice cases and fill out the **Case Study Worksheet** for each case. Some of the information will be in your reference books, some in the case studies, some already in your brain, and some you may not know—you will have to look up the definitions and meanings. This will help you move through the case smoothly and get more out of it. How much you have to look up will depend on where you are in your program, what you know, and how much experience you already have. Preparing cases will become easier as you advance in your program.

In every clinical setting, there are always things you wish you knew, but that information may not be available. That is a matter of reality—in each situation, you do the best you can with what information is provided. After a while, your instructor may tell you it is not necessary to include your **Case Study Worksheet ✓ Preparation** when you turn in your case studies unless you need to do a **Case Study Worksheet ✓ Self-Correction** as part of your self-correction assignment. After you look up the meanings, go back and underline those pieces of information in the case that seem as if they may be important. (Resist the temptation to underline everything!) Later, you will notice there are things you should have underlined or looked up, but didn't. After a few cases, you will become better at recognizing what information is relevant.

About the Sample Cases

Throughout the sample cases, you will find sentences and paragraphs marked "HINT." These are comments we have provided to help you get an idea of the kind of things you need to consider. Use them as guides to gain insight into the complexity of what appear to be very simple questions. Nothing in life is as easy or simple as it appears. This is also true of cases. However, with time, you will find yourself automatically thinking of your own "hints," whether in working through case studies, or in real clinical situations. Continually ask yourself, "How would I teach this to a student?"

If you become "stuck," try to break down the question into simpler components (analysis). See whether you can identify the relevant knowledge issues, their significance (or those things that may not be significant), and how they specifically fit into this situation (application). Look for "missing links" (as detectives call them).

There are also some sections marked "CLUE." These are extra tips, designed to help you increase your powers of observation. They can help fill in some of the "missing links."

The first case involves a teaching situation. This example integrates such problems as communication skills, knowledge of medications, vital signs skills, and using published standards and guidelines as well as the Internet to obtain professional and consumer information. The second case involves an emergency setting in which national standards are integrated into your decision making.

Throughout this book, response evaluation symbols or codes will be located in the margin next to each question. By using these to evaluate your answers, your instructor can interact with you and help you determine what kind of self-corrective measures you need to take. Then, if you continue having difficulty with an assignment, these codes can also help guide you and your instructor in identifying patterns showing where you appear to be having the most difficulty. That way, the help you get can be more focused and practical.

As you read through these cases, practice success imaging. Go through the scenario and the questions, and try to mentally picture yourself in the very scene you are reading about. Consider this as a script or a screen play. Imagine yourself asking questions, doing assessment, performing your nursing procedures, and acting out what you suggest in your answers. Picture yourself on the telephone, communicating with another nurse, a family member, or a practitioner. What do you say? What do you do?

Stop at the end of each sentence and each question. Think about what has just been said and what it means. In your mind, you need to become the star of your own movies ("Super Nurse Cheryl Strikes Again"). The more realistically you envision your interaction, the more likely you will know to do the right thing in a crisis situation later on. And keep this in mind: every case in this book, like the above stories, is reality-based, taken from honest-to-goodness, real-life nursing situations.

Finally, we want to share this with you: We (the authors and your instructors) want you to do well. We want you to be the best. It is our wish for you to grow into confident, competent professionals of whom we can be proud. After all, someday we will be one of those older people you care for and you will be the nurse in charge. When that day comes, we want you to be very, very good!

Sample Case Study 1

Name ______________________ Class/Group ______ Date ______

Group Members ______________________________________

INSTRUCTIONS: All questions apply to this case study. Your responses should be brief and to the point. Adequate space has been provided for answers. When asked to provide several answers, they should be listed in order of priority or significance. Do not assume information that is not provided. Please print or write clearly. If your response is not legible, it will be marked as ? and you will need to rewrite it.

❍ ❍ ❍ / ❍ ❍

Scenario

You have just accepted a new position as an office RN for a busy internal medicine physician. During your interviews with her, she told you that patient education was very important to her but she has found that she never has enough time to give adequate teaching. Part of your new job is to help her with patient management and education in her already established hypertension clinic.

On your first day at the hypertension clinic, you meet Mrs. M.P., a lively 78-year-old African-American woman who tells you she was told she had "hypertension" two months ago. She is 5 feet 4 inches tall and weighs 110 pounds. You take her blood pressure (BP) according to approved standards[1] and get 160/102. Her other vital signs (VS) are 78-16-98.2° F. She also tells you that the doctor told her she has to take a pill every day. As you talk with her, you notice she seems confused by her diagnosis and isn't clear about taking her medication. She asks you, "What is hypertension, anyway?"

HINT: Try to think and picture yourself through the above scenario before reading further.

HINT: Look at the **Case Study Worksheet ✓ Preparation** as you work through the next few pages to help you understand what is happening and to get hints for answering the questions. In the above paragraph, a beginner may have to look up what an "internal medicine physician" is. "Patient education," "patient management," and "hypertension" may also be terms you need to look up. A more experienced student probably will know what all those terms mean. This will give you an opportunity to expand your vocabulary and understanding of clinical settings as you think through these cases.

HINT: Many places are converting to the metric system. Practice by calculating her height and weight in centimeters and kilograms: _____ cm _______ kg

What can you learn from the above information? How many pieces of information can you count?

HINT: First you have to identify and assemble the data. Go back and look at the scenario—resist the temptation to "peek" at the next section for answers. Also, try to figure out what data in the above scenario is useful and what is not relevant to this situation.

[1] Guidelines for hypertension classification, causes, and treatment were developed by the Joint National Committee on Detection, Evaluation, and Treatment of High Blood Pressure (JNC). This Web site has instructions on the most scientifically sound way to measure blood pressures in an office setting. Search the above Internet resources to see where you can find reports by the JNC. One of the best resources for professionals is *http://www.guidelines.gov*, a site that features the JNC report reports. It also links to excellent patient-information and educational resources. Look under "diseases/conditions," and then under "cardiovascular." The JNC also has recommended lifestyle changes that nurses can discuss with patients. Use this information to answer some of the questions in this case. Remember this page—you will be able to use it to get information on many kinds of health care problems.

Information includes the following: (1) patient's age; (2) her gender; (3) the fact that she is African-American; (4) her name (referred to as "Mrs. M.P." in this case); (5) her diagnosis (always double-check this and determine whether the person is using the correct diagnostic term-sometimes people are confused about this and may tell you they have something they don't have or confuse it for something else); (6) when the diagnosis was made (2 months ago); (7) her current BP (160/102); (8) that BP was taken correctly; (9) her VS; (10) the fact that she has a prescription—an antihypertensive; and (11) the fact that she does not seem to understand or is confused by her diagnosis. These data are relevant to meaning or application questions. That is, can you take the information you have and figure out how it relates? What does the information mean? What does it tell you?

CLUE: Sometimes names can be a clue to a person's cultural orientation, but don't jump to conclusions: marriage, immigration, and adoption can mislead you. It is always important to ask how the person would prefer to be addressed. Always give the person the option of being referred to by title (Mr., Mrs. Ms., Dr., Rev., etc.).

HINT: When listening to information people tell you, be careful. You can't always assume everything they tell you is accurate. There is always the possibility the information they give us is incorrect, or they aren't telling the truth. Usually the problem is more simple (and often our fault): They are confused by the rapid-fire "big words" we throw at them. Ask them to explain things in their own words. In the case of Mrs. M.P., ask her where she heard the word "hypertension" and what she has heard about it. Remember Einstein? Sometimes you learn a lot more by asking good questions.

HINT: Patients are often anxious, intimidated, or tired. When people are anxious, they tend not to remember everything they're told (a good reason to write down the important things so they can look at it later). Ask yourself what insight these data give into the patient and their support systems, their needs, and what you need to know to provide them with good nursing care.

HINT: The incidence of hypertension increases as the population ages. Why? Some good information can be found in your pathophysiology book. You may also find valuable information at the American Heart Association Web site *http://www.americanheart.org* as well as *http://www.guidelines.gov*.

What is the significance of the knowledge that the patient is African-American? Hypertension is very common and affects approximately 20% of whites and 30% of African-Americans 18 years of age and older. You also can explain that hypertension increases with age and that 50% of all people over the age of 65 are affected. Because Mrs. M.P. is an older African-American woman, she is more likely to have hypertension than a younger woman or a white woman. On the other hand, just because a person is older doesn't automatically mean he or she will have hypertension. Also, look at Mrs. M.P.'s height and weight. We often read that obesity and hypertension are linked. Is she obese? Remember the comments about "assumptions" from the Introduction?

HINT: When you work with national standards or guidelines, always be sure you are using the most recent version. These guidelines represent recommendations based on the best scientific knowledge to date. As research shows us better ways to diagnose and treat disease, these guidelines change, so be sure you are using the most recent information. The Internet offers an invaluable service since it is possible to check for the most recent standards within a few minutes of logging on. These guidelines provide a standard for quality in measuring BP. If you have never read them, you need to get a copy and practice taking BP readings accordingly. You should also know these standards well enough to teach them to others. Professionals are responsible for maintaining high standards of practice. In another year or two, you will also be responsible for teaching and monitoring nursing assistants, students, and others as they perform these skills. BP values are very important. Because abnormal BP readings can indicate a serious problem exists, they must be accurate every time. BP measurements must be consistent and accurate, no matter who takes them. Poor BP measurement techniques are one of the most common sources of inaccurate clinical data.

What is the significance of a BP of 160/102?

HINT: Is that all the information you need to know? What about the circumstances under which it was taken? What about the environment? What about other health conditions? In addition to professional as well as public information on The American Heart Association (AHA) Web site, the National Heart, Lung, and Blood Institute (NHLBI), part of the National Institutes of Health (NIH), also has a direct Web page with standards and recommendations: *http://www.nhlbi.nih.gov/guidelines/hypertension*.

Some of these public education materials are now available in Spanish. According to information on either of the above sites, is the patient's BP considered "abnormal"? What are the therapeutic goals for someone with uncomplicated, primary hypertension (look up the difference between primary and secondary hypertension). Notice that other coexisting pathologies determine how BP is treated.

HINT: Back to Mrs. M.P.'s BP values: What is the upper (first) number called: What does it mean? What is the lower (second) number called? What does it mean? What stage of hypertension does she have? Is staging done according to the upper or the lower number?

CLUE: You have her BP as well as her other VS. Are the other VS directly relevant to this problem? It is important to learn to focus on the most significant clues.

BONUS QUESTION: If you were to take Mrs. M.P.'s BP while she was vigorously exercising on a treadmill, would a BP reading of 160 be considered abnormal? Stop and think about this before reading on. OK, we'll give you the answer this time. No, an increase in systolic BP during vigorous exercise is considered normal because it reflects increased work by the heart as it delivers more blood to working muscles. However, the diastolic BP stays about the same or may even decrease with exertion. Failure of the diastolic BP to rise during exertion may be a sign of serious heart disease.

All this was background material for the first question:

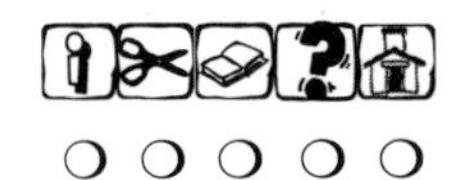

1. How would you explain hypertension to Mrs. M.P.? ❍ ❍ ❍ ❍ ❍

HINT: The first thing to consider is how to communicate in a way other persons can understand. What language do they speak? What is their educational level? What is their cultural background? How much do they already understand about their condition? Do they already know what their diagnosis means? Is their knowledge accurate? Age, sensory acuity (such as hearing or vision) and socioeconomic status are also some factors that may affect communication. Not all this information is provided in Sample Case Study 1. Part of the challenge is to discover some of this information.

HINT: When you are a student, you are learning to communicate in two new languages at once. You have to learn the language of medicine and health care—most of these words are new to you. Then you have to learn how to communicate in the language of the people you are talking with. This is a special challenge because it requires "simultaneous translation," an advanced skill among professional translators. If you look around on the NHLBI web site, you will discover some excellent patient education materials. See whether you can find professional and patient education materials about hypertension in older women.

HINT: Look at your "cheat sheet"—what is "hypertension"? How would you explain it to the patient in simple, straightforward terms?

HINT: You should start by explaining to Mrs. M.P. that hypertension (HTN) is the medical term used for high BP. Then you have to explain what BP is in simple terms and why it should be treated. Does she know what can happen when hypertension is not controlled?

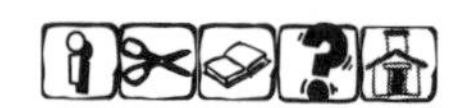

Mrs. M.P. takes a prescription pill bottle out of her purse. The label tells you it is hydrochlorothiazide (HCTZ) 12.5 mg and that 1 tablet should be taken daily for a month.

CLUE: You notice there are a lot of pills left in the bottle and it was filled over two months ago. What does that tell you?

2. You have just observed a fact (knowledge): a prescription bottle that is labeled as filled over two months ago with a lot of pills left in the bottle. There are many reasons for this besides the obvious. The obvious assumption is that she has not been taking her pills as prescribed. Some professionals would label this "noncompliance" in a way that implies that the patient is deliberately uncooperative with the treatment. That is a big assumption that may not have a basis in reality. List at least two other explanations for the fact. (Try to stretch your imagination here.) ❍ ❍ ❍ ❍ ❍

HINTS: (1) Some people will share a prescription they have sitting on the shelf with a friend "so as not to waste money" (this is dangerous as well as illegal, but many people are not aware of the danger); (2) Mrs. M.P. may have gotten the prescription filled and poured it into an older bottle (pharmacies usually place pills in "childproof" containers, but many older adults have arthritis or some other reason they can't use those containers); (3) She may not understand the importance of taking her medication every day (many people think that if they feel fine, they don't need to take their medication—this is very common in hypertension and diabetes); (4) She may have poured other pills in with the medication originally in this bottle (some people do not understand the danger of mixing different types of medication in the same container); (5) She may be forgetful (it is not easy to remember whether you have taken pills every day); (6) Sometimes people can't afford to fill their prescriptions but may be too embarrassed to say so. None of this is indicative of someone who is being deliberately uncooperative.

3. You look in the pill bottle—the pills look like the right kind and have the same markings on them. What questions would you ask Mrs. M.P. to figure out what the problem is? (Since you have read the above "HINTS," you can use them to help you formulate some of your questions.) ❍ ❍ ❍ ❍ ❍

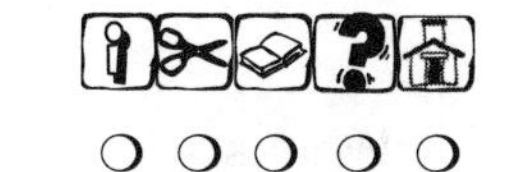

4. From the above information, there is one big clue, based on an objective measure, that indicates Mrs. M.P. may not be taking her BP medication regularly or correctly. What is it?

❍ ❍ ❍ ❍ ❍

HINT: Look at her BP reading. Does it look like it belongs to someone who is taking medication to reduce BP?

Mrs. M.P. tells you she feels just fine and doesn't think she needs to take her pills.

5. What will you tell her?

❍ ❍ ❍ ❍ ❍

HINT: Explain to Mrs. M.P. that high BP is usually asymptomatic but that treatment is essential. By explaining what hypertension can do if left untreated, you will enhance her understanding of her condition and, ideally, help with medication compliance. Start by explaining that HTN is the most significant risk factor for the development of atherosclerotic coronary artery disease (CAD). You should also explain that HTN, if left untreated, can cause damage to numerous organs but especially her eyes and her kidneys. Worst of all, HTN can lead to a cerebrovascular accident (CVA or stroke) with resulting impairment or death. For most patients, the possibility of a stroke is the most dramatic and convincing warning.

6. Mrs. M.P. also tells you the pills make her dizzy and that she has to keep getting up at night to urinate. How are you going to respond?

❍ ❍ ❍ ❍ ❍

HINT: First acknowledge the legitimacy of her complaints. Falling (from dizziness) and disturbed sleep can create more serious problems.

7. What self-care tips can you share with Mrs. M.P. that may help with the side effects of her medication?

HINT: Show her how to get up from a supine or seated position slowly and safely. Alcohol intake can also make a person more subject to falls. Suggest she take the pill in the morning rather than in the evening so her sleep is less disturbed. Falls at night when people are sleepy and visibility is worse can be very serious for anyone, especially the elderly who have poorer sensory perception and balance.

8. You have the receptionist schedule Mrs. M.P. to return in a month for a reevaluation office visit. Upon what do you base the decision to have her return in a month rather than a shorter or longer period?

HINT: The JNC guidelines provide the framework for determining follow-up. The most recent JNC report has a table with this information.

9. What arrangements could you make with Mrs. M.P. to encourage her to take her medication? (Keep in mind, you also need to monitor to see whether this is the correct medication for her.)

HINT: (1) Give her a wallet-sized card on which she can record her BP measurements at least once a week; (2) Ask whether she lives near a fire station, a senior citizens' center, or some place where her BP can be checked at least once a week at the same time of day. If she lives near your office, encourage her to stop by for free BP checks at least once a week; (3) Telephone follow-up calls are a good way to determine how she is doing and to get feedback. Make an appointment to call her at a specific time to encourage her.

10. Frequently, it may be necessary to try several medications to find the one that works best and has side-effects that are acceptable to the individual. (This is highly individualized.) Where did you find guidelines concerning which medications should be tested in what order? Is Mrs. M.P. taking one of those recommended medications? ❍ ❍ ❍ ❍ ❍

HINT: Again, the JNC guidelines suggest which types of medications should be used in various populations.

Mrs. M.P. tells you her mother died of a stroke at the same age she is now. She says she is "scared to death" the same thing will happen to her. You share with Mrs. M.P. that federal guidelines recommend a BP goal of less than 140/90 (for non-diabetic patients). You tell her that you will be glad to work together with her to achieve the recommended level. She thanks you for explaining everything to her and reports she will get her prescription filled today on the way home from the doctor's office.

For the next three weeks, you call Mrs. M.P. every Thursday before lunch. She tells you she has been taking her pill every morning and has been having her BP at the senior center. She reports her weekly BP as "154 and 92," "148 and 90," and "148 and 92."

Mrs. M.P. returns to the office for her next appointment. She sits down to get her BP taken and tells you she has been doing everything you taught her. When you ask her whether she has any questions, she says "No."

HINT: When people say they have no questions or that they remember what you taught them, do not assume that they understand or remember anything. Ask specific questions so that you know what they know. Have them try to explain it back to you in their own words.

11. You are getting ready to take Mrs. M.P.'s BP. What are important factors to keep in mind to guarantee an accurate reading? ❍ ❍ ❍ ❍ ❍

HINT: Refer to the JNC guidelines to fill this in.

12. Referring back to the JNC guidelines, would you say Mrs. M.P.'s BP is being controlled by her current medication? ❍ ❍ ❍ ❍ ❍

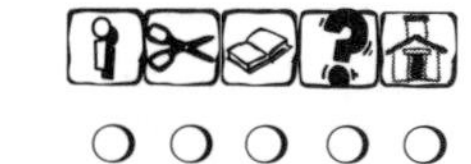

13. As part of your job, you will be putting together a patient-information library about cardiovascular related problems and interventions. Where will you find resources?

HINT: You already found two of the best, inexpensive resources on the Internet in the first questions of this case. Did you notice that the Web sites you visited had materials for patients/consumers as well as for professionals? These are extremely high-quality materials. As you can see, things you learn in one question can be used to answer other questions.

In this case, you have learned a lot of new material. For example, you have learned about educational materials, national standards or guidelines, and important skills; you have also discovered some ways to use the Internet to get supportive information, enhanced your awareness of communication issues, learned details about some medications and their side effects, enlarged your vocabulary, and much more. In other words, working on cases forces you to learn and integrate much more information than you could if you just memorized a bunch of facts. It also gives you an idea how information fits together in practice. Just as in real life, you soon will be seeing this same patient in another chapter. That case (Chapter 2, Case 1) will build on what you learned from this one.

For now, go back through the entire case. Re-read each section, then close your eyes and imagine yourself in the role of the nurse. Make a "mind video" of yourself in this situation, thinking through what you would say, what you would do, and why. As the saying goes, "Make it Yours."

Take a deep breath and congratulate yourself. You deserve it. This was a case with many details. There is no such thing as an "easy" case; each one forces you to learn a lot in a short amount of time. It's understandable that you won't get everything correct. In fact, you may get only a few questions right the first time; with more experience, you may get half right the first time around. You're allowed to get things wrong if you learn how to correct yourself. In the meanwhile, you don't have to worry—you can't harm a paper patient!

Case Study Worksheet: ✓ Preparation ___ Self-Correction

Sample

Name: ______________ Chapter 1 Case 1 Date ______________
Patient initials M.P.

Symbols/terms/abbreviations	Meaning/definition (diagnoses and medications go in following sections)

Diagnoses/medical conditions (+current and –past)	Description/meaning of diagnosis or medical problem (include possible significance)

Medications (brand and generic name if applicable)	Class, indications, contraindications, significant side effects, food and drug interactions

Treatments, interventions and therapeutic procedures	Method of delivery, purpose/desired outcome, indications, contra-indications, and precautions (Include supplemental oxygen, tube feedings, therapeutic beds, etc.)

Laboratory tests and diagnostic procedures	What is it, when was it done, and why?

Cultural issues and their significance:

Notes:

Self-Correction—Process Worksheet

The second sample case study will introduce the **Self-Correction—Process Worksheet** (found in Appendix C). This exercise will help you take feedback about your case study answers from your instructor and incorporate this feedback into corrections you will make before resubmitting. Learning by correcting your own work is more difficult than being spoon-fed corrections by an instructor, but it is a more powerful learning stimulus—and you tend to remember it.

Case Study Evaluation Codes—Process Review

The symbols or codes for each question are as follows:

1. If an answer has no box checked in the margin, it means your answer is fine as is.
2. If an answer is marked , it means the response has insufficient information. Reevaluate and rewrite to include updated or additional information.
3. If an answer is marked , it means the response is too wordy or has extra but irrelevant material. It needs to be rewritten in a more concise and focused manner.
4. If an answer is marked , it means the response is vague and difficult to understand. Rewrite the question, asking yourself what information is requested. Try to be as focused and specific as possible.
5. If an answer is marked , it means that the response is indecipherable. Rewrite it so that it can be understood.
6. This symbol is for faculty/instructors. It means that during the grading/evaluation process, nearly everyone missed something or that something related to that particular question was apparently not clear. As instructors, we all would like to think we're being perfectly clear but we get a reality orientation when we start to look at tests, papers, and other means of feed back. This symbol means this part of the case and related supportive information needs to be reviewed in class so that all can benefit from the feedback. We realize students should not be penalized when we fail to communicate well.

The **Case Study Worksheet ✓ Preparation** form is to help you condense your preparation onto a single "cheat sheet." If you need to correct a case, use the **Self-Correction—Process Worksheet** form and clip it to your resubmitted case. This helps your instructor identify whether you have assembled the factual material that is relevant to the case.

Each time you submit a case to your instructor or facilitator, one of four responses may be marked at the top of the first page. These responses and their meanings are as follows:

This indicates that your written responses indicate sound and creative thinking based on authoritative information sources. No one is perfect all the time, so you can be a rocket scientist and still need to review one or two responses marked or to try to understand why that response was questioned. Your answers and reasoning in most or all of the questions reflect problem-solving responses that a good nurse would make. Your instructor or facilitator may include a briefly worded hint or tip. You do not have to revise and resubmit your case, but please review faculty responses or class review comments on your own to learn what you did well—and where and what you can improve. Congratulate yourself on a job well done! This work is not easy. You are not expected to be perfect, nor should you expect yourself to be perfect. The goal of critical thinking and case studies is to learn how to self-learn in reality-based situations.

Good thinker: Your written responses indicate overall good thinking based on solid information sources. Please review questions marked as , , , or to identify areas for improvement. You do not have to revise and resubmit your case, but please review faculty responses on your own to learn what you did well as much as where you can improve. Congratulate yourself. This work is not easy. You are not expected to be perfect, nor should you expect yourself to be perfect. The goal of critical thinking and case studies is to learn how to self-learn in reality-based situations.

This means a question/problem needs more work. Please review, rework, and resubmit. Attach your original **Case Study Worksheet ✓ Preparation** and the **Self-Correction—Process Worksheet** to your Case Study so that your instructors or facilitator can see where you may be having problems.

(Please staple; do not fold pages, tear corners, or clip papers together.) Please review questions marked as , , , or to identify areas for improvement. Review any additional faculty responses *on your own* to learn what you did well and where you can improve. Do not be discouraged. If you did well on even a few questions, this is not a "consolation prize"—it is something to celebrate.

This means that you did well on your reworking of that question. This work is not easy. You are not expected to be perfect. The goal of critical thinking and case studies is to learn how to learn, not to be perfect in everything the first time. The good news is that by resubmitting, you still have a chance to earn an A or B. If you still have trouble in solving this study, make an appointment with your instructor or facilitator to analyze why and where you are having difficulty. Take in all your papers and notes, along with any additional questions so that your instructor can better understand. All of this is meant to help you creatively learn, not to be punishment. Someday you will be a professional nurse—part of professionalism is to learn continually and to improve the quality of your thinking processes and patient/consumer care.

This means make an appointment to see your instructor. Don't worry—this is not the Spanish Inquisition. It is an opportunity for your instructor to meet with you for individualized help to find where you think you are having trouble. This also helps the instructor learn different approaches to teaching that may help in the future. You see, instructors learn too. They need feedback on where they may have explained something better in class, or what they can do for students in the future to improve the quality of their help. Believe it or not, instructors want you to succeed. Your success helps them feel good, too!

Being asked to rework a case study is not meant to be punishment, nor should you be embarrassed by it. This process is intended to help you rethink through your assignment and document your thought processes. It is also meant to help you with self-correction and self-improvement. We all need the freedom to learn from our mistakes, and this is best done when we have the opportunity to analyze what we ourselves have done. The **Case Study Worksheet ✓ Self-Correction** form can help you identify and clarify issues related to patient care. Use it as a practice/background form to help you prepare any or all assignments.

As you fill out the form, it is a good idea to include references to help you remember where you got the material; for example "Lecture notes, date", "(Author) Med/Surg Book, page __ ", (Author) Drug Handbook, page __", "*http://www.WebPageAddress*." Remember, though, to use *current* references—outdated references can be dangerous in terms of patient care, and they lead you to learn the incorrect things.

Noting your references is important for four reasons: (1) It reminds you where you found the background information upon which to build your case studies; (2) It helps the instructor know whether you are using the best resources for your learning process; (3) It may identify sources of error upon which you based your responses; (4) It helps you increase your efficiency in identifying the best resources for use in developing your decision-making processes. You may be surprised to know that textbooks can have mistakes in them—just because something is published in a book doesn't make it absolute or true. Ask your instructor whether he or she will let you earn "bonus points" for discovering errors or discrepancies in reference books.

Do Instructors Ever Make Mistakes?

None of us is perfect. How do you communicate with your instructors or facilitators if you think they have been unfair in evaluating your work or you think you found a mistake in study materials? The way *not* to do it is to start an argument in class. This is unproductive for everyone concerned (and bad practice for real life). Instead, briefly write out where you disagree, include your reasons and documentation (see above paragraph), and submit this to the instructor prior to the next class. This gives him or her the option of discussing confusing points in class or giving you any additional points you deserve. On the other hand, if you are incorrect, it keeps you from being embarrassed in front of your classmates.

Important Notes

Clarity is critical: Your submitted work must be legible. From now on, the lives and well-being of human beings will depend on your ability to accurately and clearly communicate. Effective verbal and written communication is critical in inter- and intraprofessional relationships. If information cannot be read, it will be assumed to be incorrect. It is not the job of faculty members to try to interpret sloppy or vague work. This works both ways: It is important that you ask your instructor if you don't understand something he or she has written or if you think something is vague.

Working in groups is a helpful part of learning for most people. In addition, teamwork reflects the reality of health care. However, for all members of the group to benefit, everyone must participate and come prepared to group meetings. Copying answers from anyone, whether you received them verbally or in written form, is cheating. Remember, you are not cheating the faculty, nor are you fooling them; you are cheating yourself, your classmates/colleagues, and your future patients. In real life, there are always the few who want to depend on the hard work of others. Complaining about this to the instructor will not help. The best solution is for the group to confront the individual. In group assignments, individuals who do not prepare and who depend on others for their answers should be asked by the group to "do the work or leave." This is not the job of faculty; it is yours, and it is part of preparation for professional practice. You engage in faculty and class evaluation as part of your responsibility now. This is a serious process. In a short time, you will be a practicing professional who will be asked to evaluate supervisors/managers, peers, assistive personnel, and students. If you want to be treated and evaluated fairly, you must do the same for others. This is not an easy process to learn, but you can start practicing this now.

Sample Case Study 2

Name ______________________ Class/Group ______ Date ______

Group Members ______________________________________

INSTRUCTIONS: All questions apply to this case study. Your responses should be brief and to the point. Adequate space has been provided for answers. When asked to provide several answers, they should be listed in order of priority or significance. Do not assume information that is not provided. Please print or write clearly. If your response is not legible, it will be marked as ? and you will need to rewrite it.

❍ ❍ ❍ / ❍ ❍

Scenario

You are the nurse on duty in an extended care facility. At suppertime, you enter a patient's room and find her unconscious and not breathing. The patient's meal tray is in front of her, and a quick glance tells you there is a part of an orange on it.

HINT: As you become more experienced, you will learn to concentrate in emergencies. You will learn to absorb quickly the important clues in a situation.

1. What is the first action you should take? ❍ ❍ ❍ ❍ ❍

The patient does not respond.

2. What should you do next? ❍ ❍ ❍ ❍ ❍

3. How would you open the airway? ❍ ❍ ❍ ❍ ❍

The patient is not breathing.

4. What are your next actions?

After attempting rescue breathing, the patient's chest does not rise.

5. What should you do next?

You detect no obstruction.

6. What should you do next?

After repeated maneuvers, the situation remains unchanged.

7. What should your next action be?

The paramedics arrive and attempt to ventilate the patient manually with a bag-valve mask device. They are unable to ventilate the patient's lungs. Next they attempt to intubate the patient. While visualizing with the laryngoscope, a paramedic notices dentures and a piece of orange in the patient's airway.

8. How could this obstruction have occurred? ❍ ❍ ❍ ❍ ❍

The obstructions are removed, the patient is intubated, manually ventilated, and transported to the hospital. She suffers a cardiac arrest in the ambulance, and all attempts to resuscitate are unsuccessful. The patient is pronounced dead on arrival at the hospital.

9. List at least three steps that could have been taken in this scenario that may have averted this outcome. List preventive measures first. ❍ ❍ ❍ ❍ ❍

10. Where did you get the information you included in your response to question 9? What is your source? Check the resources you used in Sample Case Study 1. Did you use the most recent versions of the standards? ❍ ❍ ❍ ❍ ❍

Good job! Now go back and review what you have written. Think it through. Go over the material, question by question, either in class or in a group. Pretend you are the instructor, and underline the things you need to improve or correct. Evaluate your answers, using the coded check boxes at the right of each question. Be tough with yourself. Next, use the **Self-Correction—Process Worksheet** and reevaluate your responses, writing the answers in the appropriate blanks. Think through why you made a mistake and try to understand what you would do differently next time. (For your convenience, suggested answers for this case are provided on the following page.)

Did you recognize the scenario in Sample Case Study 2? This case gave you the chance to take information you have learned from your past and apply it to a current problem. This is mostly an application case; it requires you to bring facts to play, understand their significance, and apply them to the scenario. When you review the case for accuracy, you are using the process of analysis to check your own answers and figure out what needs to be corrected.

Now read through from the beginning of the case and make your "mind movie." Think through, step by step, what you would do in this setting if you had to repeat it. Remember, as the nurse, you are in a decision-making position. Your actions will have a powerful influence on people's lives.

Case Study Worksheet: _✓_ Preparation ___ Self-Correction

Sample

Name: ______________________ Chapter __1__ Case __2__ Date __________

Patient initials _______

Symbols/terms/abbreviations	Meaning/definition (diagnoses and medications go in following sections)
______________	______________________________
______________	______________________________
______________	______________________________
______________	______________________________
______________	______________________________
______________	______________________________
______________	______________________________
______________	______________________________

Diagnoses/medical conditions (+current and –past)	Description/meaning of diagnosis or medical problem (include possible significance)
______________	______________________________
	______________________________
______________	______________________________
	______________________________
______________	______________________________
	______________________________
______________	______________________________
	______________________________
______________	______________________________
	______________________________

Medications (brand and generic name if applicable)	Class, indications, contraindications, significant side effects, food and drug interactions
______________	______________________________
	______________________________
______________	______________________________
	______________________________
______________	______________________________
	______________________________
______________	______________________________
	______________________________
______________	______________________________
	______________________________

Treatments, interventions and therapeutic procedures	Method of delivery, purpose/desired outcome, indications, contraindications, and precautions (Include supplemental oxygen, tube feedings, therapeutic beds, etc.)
______	______
______	______
______	______
______	______
______	______
______	______

Laboratory tests and diagnostic procedures	What is it, when was it done, and why?
______	______
______	______
______	______
______	______
______	______
______	______
______	______
______	______
______	______
______	______

Cultural issues and their significance:

______
______
______
______
______
______

Notes:

Permission for unrestricted number of copies of this form may be made for use in conjunction with this book and corresponding clinical use by legitimate owners of this book only.

Self-Correction—Process Worksheet

Name: ______________________ Chapter _____ Case _____ Date ___________

Questions revised on this worksheet: ___, ___, ___, ___, ___

Question # ___ ❍ ❍ ❍ ❍ ❍

Revision: ____

Question # ___ ❍ ❍ ❍ ❍ ❍

Revision: ____

Question # ___ ❍ ❍ ❍ ❍ ❍

Revision: ____

❍ ❍ ❍ ❍ ❍

Question # ___

Revision: ___

❍ ❍ ❍ ❍ ❍

Question # ___

Revision: ___

Overall evaluation: ❍ ❍ ❍ / ❍ ❍

Additional feedback from instructor: ___

Permission for unrestricted number of copies of this form may be made for use in conjunction with this book and corresponding clinical use by legitimate owners of this book only.

Suggested Answers for Sample Case Study 2

1. What is the first action you should take?

 - The first action you take will depend on what you already know. You should always know the current code status of each patient. If this patient has DNR (Do Not Resuscitate) orders, then you do *not* resuscitate. You let her go, clean her body, and notify the family and the attending physician.
 - If she is in full code, establish unresponsiveness by shaking the patient gently and asking, "Are you okay?"

2. What would you do next?

 - Open the airway and check for breathing.

3. How would you open the airway?

 - Jaw thrust, chin lift.

4. What are your next actions?

 - Give two deep breaths.
 - Call a code or dial 911 if you are not equipped to handle an emergency.

5. What should you do next?

 - Perform blind finger sweep to attempt to remove a possible obstruction.
 - Do not do this if the patient is seizing.

6. What should you do next?

 - Proceed with the Heimlich maneuver for an unconscious victim.

7. What should your next action be?

 - Attempt ventilations again, and repeat the Heimlich maneuver until obstruction is dislodged.

8. How could this obstruction have occurred?

 - The patient could have aspirated them herself.

9. What three steps could have been taken in this scenario that may have averted this outcome? List preventive measures first.

 - Don't give an elderly person large pieces of fruit. Serve fruit in small pieces.
 - Make sure patients receiving solid food are able to chew and swallow safely—and that their dentures fit well.
 - Always check the throat for dentures in a nonbreathing victim if you cannot find them.
 - Always LOOK into the airway of an unconscious, nonbreathing victim.

10. Where did you get the information you included in your response to question 9? What is your source? Check the resources you used in Sample Case Study 1. Did you use the most recent version of the standards?

- The American Heart Association has published guidelines. These are what you learned when you obtained your CPR (cardiopulmonary resuscitation) certification. The protocol, or standards you followed, were categorized as "Adult Foreign Body Airway Obstruction—Unconscious."
- Guidelines change, so be sure to check the most recent date of change.

That should give you an idea of how to work through the cases in this book. Of course, each case is different, but the step-by-step, learn-to-correct-yourself approach will not change.

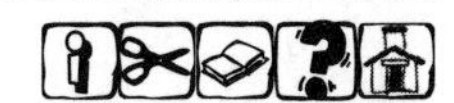

Bonus problem: Remind Mrs. M.P. that she should continue with her prescribed medications and not make any alterations. Especially emphasize the need to talk with you or the physician before she starts taking any "natural" or herbal remedies, over-the-counter remedies for cold or flu, or nutritional supplements. Name one herbal remedy or natural product that could elevate her BP.

Case Study 3

Name ______________________ Class/Group ______ Date ______

Group Members ______________________________________

INSTRUCTIONS: All questions apply to this case study. Your responses should be brief and to the point. Adequate space has been provided for answers. When asked to provide several answers, they should be listed in order of priority or significance. Do not assume information that is not provided. Please print or write clearly. If your response is not legible, it will be marked as ? and you will need to rewrite it.

Scenario

You are a nurse at a free-standing cardiac prevention and rehabilitation center. Your new client in risk-factor modification is B.J., a 37-year-old traveling salesman, who is married and has 3 children. During a recent evaluation for chest pain (including a cardiac catheterization), he was diagnosed with angina pectoris, given a prescription for SL nitroglycerin, told how to use it, and referred to your cardiac rehabilitation program for sessions 3 days a week. B.J.'s wife comes along to help him with healthy lifestyle changes. You take the following nursing history: B.J.'s father died of sudden cardiac death at age 42, and his mother (still living) had a CABG x 4 (quadruple coronary artery bypass graft) at age 52; his hypertension is controlled with nifedipine (Procardia) 90 mg PO qd, which he has taken regularly; he has averaged 1½ cigarette packs per day for 20 years; an "occasional" beer ("a 6-pack every weekend with the football game"*); and a dietary history of fried and fast foods. His current weight is 235 at 5'8"; he has a waist circumference of 48 inches. His VS are 138/88, 82, 18, 98.4° F.

Note: Be alert to the fact that many individuals tend to underreport their alcohol and drug consumption. Clearly mark patient reports by using quotes to indicate subjective source of information.

1. Calculate B.J.'s smoking history in terms of pack-years.

2. List three nonmodifiable risk factors for CAD.

3. List six modifiable risk factors for CAD.

4. Underline each of the responses in questions 1 and 2 that represent B.J.'s personal CAD risk factors.

5. You would like to know more about B.J.'s hyperlipidemia. What 4 common laboratory values do you need to know?

B.J. laughingly tells you he believes in the 5 all-American food groups: salt, sugar, fat, chocolate, and caffeine.

6. Identify health-related problems in this case description; the problem that is potentially life-threatening should be listed first.

7. Of all his behaviors, which one is the most significant in promoting cardiac disease?

8. What is the most important priority problem that you need to address with B.J.? Identify the teaching strategy you would use with him.

HINT: What *you* think is the most important may not be what *he* considers the most important, or the one he is willing to work on.

9. What is the second problem you would work with B.J. to change? Identify an appropriate strategy to resolve the problem.

Note: Whenever B.J. and his wife decide to attack dietary changes, try to get a referral to an RD who can work with them to develop palatable meals and do long-term planning. Many more states are requiring registration of dietitians in the same way nurses are registered. Check to make certain that dietary counseling for a person with specific disease states is not exceeding the nursing standard of practice for your state.

10. B.J.'s wife takes you aside and tells you, "I'm so worried for B. I grew up in a really dysfunctional family where there was a lot of violence. B. has been so good to the kids and me. I'm so worried I'll lose him that I have nightmares about his heart stopping. I find myself suddenly awakening at night just to see if he's breathing." How are you going to respond?

Note: Nightmares about losing a loved one to heart disease are not rare, especially during the time of diagnosis or disease-related crisis. However, a background of childhood violence can have deep roots and often requires special help. Clearly, this woman is in distress. Depending on her willingness at this time, it would be good for her to talk with a therapist. If she doesn't think she needs it, try suggesting that it might be good for B.J. and the kids and that it would help her relax and be more responsive to them. At the appropriate point, it would be important for her to be able to share with her husband how she feels. From her description, this sleep disturbance is an unhealthy situation that should be addressed. If she refuses, keep an open relationship; it is important that she keep talking to someone about her fear.

Six weeks after you start working with B.J., he admits that he has been under a lot of stress. He rubs his chest and says, "It feels really heavy on my chest right now." You feel his pulse and note that his skin is slightly diaphoretic, and that he is agitated and appears to be very anxious.

11. What are you going to do to obtain additional information? ❍ ❍ ❍ ❍ ❍

12. B.J. continues to feel symptomatic. Now what are you going to do? ❍ ❍ ❍ ❍ ❍

Case Study 4

Name ______________________ Class/Group ______ Date ______

Group Members ______________________________________

INSTRUCTIONS: All questions apply to this case study. Your responses should be brief and to the point. Adequate space has been provided for answers. When asked to provide several answers, they should be listed in order of priority or significance. Do not assume information that is not provided. Please print or write clearly. If your response is not legible, it will be marked as ? and you will need to rewrite it.

❍ ❍ ❍ / ❍ ❍

Scenario

J.F. is a 50-year-old married homemaker with a genetic autoimmune deficiency; she has suffered from recurrent bacterial endocarditis. The most recent episodes were a *Staphylococcus aureus* infection of the mitral valve 16 months ago and a *Streptococcus mutans* infection of the aortic valve 1 month ago. During this latter hospitalization, an echocardiogram showed aortic stenosis, moderate aortic insufficiency, chronic valvular vegetations, and moderate atrial enlargement. Two years ago J.F. received an 18-month course of TPN therapy for malnutrition caused by idiopathic, relentless nausea and vomiting (N/V). She has also had CAD for several years, and 2 years ago suffered an acute anterior wall MI. In addition, she has a history of chronic joint pain.

Now, after being home for only a week, J.F. has been readmitted to your floor with endocarditis, N/V, and renal failure. Since yesterday she has been vomiting and retching constantly; she also has had chills, fever, fatigue, joint pain, and headache. As you go through the admission process with her, you note that she wears glasses and has a dental bridge. She is immediately started on TPN at 125 ml/h and on penicillin 2 million units IV q4h, to be continued for 4 weeks. Other medications are furosemide 80 mg PO qd, amiodipine 5 mg PO qd, K-Dur 40 mEq PO qd (dose adjusted according to laboratory results), metoprolol 25 mg PO bid, and droperidol 0.25–0.5 ml IVP prn for N/V. Admission VS are 152/48 (supine) and 100/40 (sitting), 116, 22, 37.9° C. When you assess her, you find a grade II/VI holosystolic murmur and a grade III/VI diastolic murmur; 2+ pitting tibial edema but no peripheral cyanosis; clear lungs; orientation x 3 but drowsy; soft abdomen with slight LUQ tenderness; hematuria; and multiple petechiae on skin of arms, legs, and chest.

1. What is the significance of the orthostatic hypotension, the wide pulse pressure, and the tachycardia? ❍ ❍ ❍ ❍ ❍

2. What is the significance of the abdominal tenderness, hematuria, joint pain, and petechiae? ❍ ❍ ❍ ❍ ❍

3. As you monitor J.F. throughout the day, what other s/s of embolization will you watch for?

4. Three important diagnostic criteria for infectious endocarditis are anemia, fever, and cardiac murmurs. Explain the cause for each sign.

5. On the day after admission, you review J.F.s laboratory test results: Na 138 mmol/L, K 3.9 mmol/L, Cl 103 mmol/L, BUN 85 mg/dL, creatinine 3.9 mg/dL, glucose 185 mg/dL, WBCs 6.7 thou/cmm, Hct 27%, Hgb 9.0 g/dL. Identify the values that are not within normal ranges, and explain the reason for each abnormality.

6. Which laboratory value(s) reflect(s) catabolism of muscle, and what does muscle catabolism accomplish?

7. If the TPN is scheduled on a 24-hour basis, when would blood glucose be drawn, and why?

8. Why would blood glucose monitoring be important?

9. What is the greatest risk for J.F. during the process of rehydration, and what would you monitor to detect its development?

As you admitted J.F., you were aware that as soon as she became stable, she would be going home in a few days on TPN and IV antibiotics. The home care agency that will be supervising her care is contacted to coordinate discharge preparations and teaching as soon as possible.

10. List five important questions in assessing her home health care needs.

Fortunately, J.F. has a supportive husband and 2 daughters who live nearby who can function as caregivers when J.F. is discharged. They, as well as the patient, will also need teaching about endocarditis. Although J.F. has been ill for several years, you discover that she and her family have received little education about the disease. You prepare a teaching plan for the family. The home care agency has a PEN-team (parenteral enteral nutrition team) to address her nutritional needs, which will also include vitamins, minerals, and lipids. TPN formulations require complex calculations. The PEN-team takes care of the formulation of the TPN through the pharmacy or dietary staff (depending on local arrangements).

11. List two predisposing causes of bacteremia that you will explain.

12. List three other things you would teach.

Your hospital discharge planner facilitates J.F.'s transition to home care.

13. During the initial home visit, the home health nurse evaluates J.F.'s IV site for implementation of the IV therapy program. The nurse interviews the family members to determine their willingness to be caregivers and their level of understanding and enlists the patient's and family's assistance to identify 10 teaching goals. What topics would be included on this list?

14. The home health nurse also writes short- and long-term goals for J.F. and her family. Identify two short-term and three long-term goals.

    Short-term goals

    Long-term goals

Mr. F. and his 2 daughters learned to administer J.F.'s TPN during the 18-month treatment. Be aware that IV cases are usually covered by most insurers on a case-by-case basis and with clear documentation.

15. What documentation would be required in order to obtain reimbursement? (Need to clearly document everything that is done and why, in detail.)

Case Study 5

Name ________________________ Class/Group ______ Date ______

Group Members ______________________________________

INSTRUCTIONS: All questions apply to this case study. Your responses should be brief and to the point. Adequate space has been provided for answers. When asked to provide several answers, they should be listed in order of priority or significance. Do not assume information that is not provided. Please print or write clearly. If your response is not legible, it will be marked as ? and you will need to rewrite it.

❍ ❍ ❍ / ❍ ❍

Scenario

It is midmorning on the cardiac unit where you work, and you are getting a new patient. G.P., a 60-year-old retired businessman, is married and has 3 grown children. As you take his health history, he tells you that he began feeling changes in his heart rhythm about 10 days ago. He has hypertension and a 5-year history of angina pectoris. During the past week he has had more frequent episodes of midchest discomfort. The chest pain has awakened him from sleep but does respond to NTG, which he has taken sublingually about 8 to 10 times over the past week. During the week he has also experienced increased fatigue. He states, "I just feel crappy all the time anymore." A cardiac catheterization done several years ago revealed 50% occlusion of the right coronary artery (RCA) and 50% occlusion of the left anterior descending (LAD) coronary artery. He tells you that both his mother and father had CAD. He is taking amlodipine, metoprolol, lipitor, and baby ASA qd.

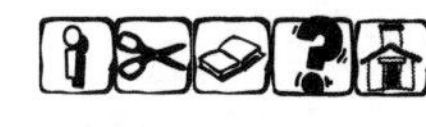

1. What other information are you going to ask about his episodes of chest pain? ❍ ❍ ❍ ❍ ❍

2. What are common sites for radiation of ischemic cardiac pain? ❍ ❍ ❍ ❍ ❍

Note: Patients will tell you what you want to hear, so be careful how you ask your questions.

3. You know that G.P. has atherosclerosis of the coronary arteries but he has not told you about his risk factors. You need to know his risk factors for CAD in order to plan teaching for lifestyle modifications. What will you ask him about?

4. Although he has been taking SL NTG for a long time, you want to be sure he is using it correctly. What information would you make sure he understands about the side effects, use, and storage of sublingual NTG?

When you first admitted G.P., you placed him on telemetry and observed he was in A fib converting frequently to atrial flutter with a 4:1 block. His VS and all of his lab tests were within normal range, including troponin and CK levels; K was 4.7 mmol/L. He was converted with medications (quinidine and diltiazem) from A fib/atrial flutter to tachy/brady syndrome with long sinus pauses that caused lightheadedness and hypotension.

5. What risks does the new rhythm pose for G.P.?

Because G.P.'s dysrhythmia is causing unacceptable symptoms, he is taken to surgery and a permanent DDI pacemaker is placed and set at a rate of 70/minute.

6. What does the code "DDI" mean?

7. The pacemaker insertion surgery places G.P. at risk for several serious complications. List three potential problems that you will monitor for as you care for him.

8. G.P. will need some education regarding his new pacemaker. What information will you give him before he leaves the hospital?

Note: Information about the Medic Alert emergency identification system can be obtained by calling 1-800-432-5378.

9. G.P.'s wife approaches you and anxiously inquires, "My neighbor saw this science fiction movie about this guy who got a pacemaker and then he couldn't die. Is that for real?" How are you going to respond to her?

10. G.P. and his wife tell you they have heard that people with pacemakers can have their hearts stop because of theft and security sensors in stores and airports. Where can you help them find more information?

After discharge, G.P. is referred to a cardiac prevention and rehabilitation center to start an exercise program. He will be exercise-tested, and an individualized exercise prescription will be developed for him based on the exercise test.

11. What information will be obtained from the graded exercise (stress) test (GXT), and what is included in an exercise prescription?

Case Study 6

Name ______________________ Class/Group ______ Date ______

Group Members ____

INSTRUCTIONS: All questions apply to this case study. Your responses should be brief and to the point. Adequate space has been provided for answers. When asked to provide several answers, they should be listed in order of priority or significance. Do not assume information that is not provided. Please print or write clearly. If your response is not legible, it will be marked as ? and you will need to rewrite it.

❍ ❍ ❍ / ❍ ❍

Scenario

Mrs. R.K. is an 85-year-old woman who lives with her husband, 87. Two nights before her admission to your cardiac unit, she awoke with heavy, substernal pressure accompanied by epigastric distress. The pain was reduced somewhat when she rolled onto her side but did not completely subside for about 6 hours. The next night she experienced the same chest pressure. The following morning, Mrs. R.K.'s husband took her to the doctor and she was subsequently hospitalized to rule out (R/O) myocardial infarction (R/O MI).

Labs were drawn in the ED. She was started on O_2 2L/nc and given nonenteric coated ASA 325 mg. An IV was started.

You obtain the following information from your nursing history and physical exam: Mrs. R.K. has no history of smoking or alcohol use; has been in good general health with the exception of osteoarthritis of her hands and knees and some osteoarthritis of the spine. Her only medications are ranitidine, ibuprofen for bone and joint pain, and "herbs." Her admission VS are 132/84, 88, 18, 37.2° C. Her weight is 52 kg and height is 163 cm. Moderate edema of both ankles is present, but capillary refill and peripheral pulses are 1+. You hear a soft systolic murmur. You place her on telemetry, which shows frequent PACs but no ventricular ectopy. She denies any discomfort at present.

1. Give at least two reasons an IV would be inserted. What kind of IV fluid would you expect to be running and at what rate? ❍ ❍ ❍ ❍ ❍
(This question requires a series of mental steps: First, you need to gather your facts, then you need to figure out what they mean. You need to analyze this context, then decide what is appropriate to use.)

2. Why is "nonenteric coated" ASA specified? What would be a contraindication to administering ASA? ❍ ❍ ❍ ❍ ❍

3. Mrs. R.K. becomes fatigued during the admission process and you decide to let her sleep. When she awakens, what additional history and physical information should you obtain r/t her admitting diagnosis?

   History

   Physical Exam

4. List seven lab/diagnostic tests you would expect were drawn or conducted in the ED; suggest what each may contribute.

5. What other source, besides cardiac, may be responsible for her chest and abdominal discomfort (specify)?

❍ ❍ ❍ ❍ ❍

6. Differentiate between pain of cardiac origin and that of noncardiac origin. Be aware that little research has differentiated between the clinical symptoms experienced by women versus those experienced by men.

❍ ❍ ❍ ❍ ❍

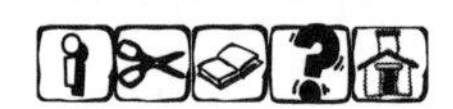

Differentiating Between Women's and Men's Cardiac-Related Symptoms

Men (more traditional "textbook" symptoms)	Women and Older Adults (may be more subtle and often attributed to other causes)
Sudden pressure, fullness, squeezing or pain in the center of the chest that is constant or intermittent	Tightness in chest, sometimes in left arm or into the jaw, sometimes mistaken for indigestion
Pain radiating from the center of the chest to the shoulders, neck, or arms	Nocturnal dyspnea or chronic breathlessness
Sudden-onset tachycardia	Dizziness, lightheadedness—etiology unknown, sometimes loss of consciousness
Perspiration, nausea, SOB, lightheadedness, chest discomfort	Chronic fatigue—unusual and overwhelming, usually worse in the evening
	Lower extremity edema (dependent), usually worse in the evening
	Heart "flutters" or palpitations
	Nausea or gastric upset (often similar to symptoms of dyspepsia or GERD)

7. Define the concept *differential diagnosis.* ❍ ❍ ❍ ❍ ❍

8. Explain how the concept of differential diagnosis applies to Mrs. R.K.'s symptoms. ❍ ❍ ❍ ❍ ❍

9. Florence Nightingale frequently emphasized the value of good observation skills in nurses. Explain how a good nursing assessment can contribute to understanding the cause of her symptoms.

10. Abnormalities on Mrs. R.K.'s 12-lead ECG were reported as "slight left axis deviation." Serial CKs are 27 U/mL, 24 U/mL, 26 U/mL; troponin is 1.1 μg/L. A series of tests R/O a noncardiac cause for her chest pain. On the basis of the information presented so far, do you believe she has had an MI? What is your rationale?

11. While you care for Mrs. R.K., you carefully observe her. Identify two possible complications of CAD and the signs and symptoms (s/s) associated with each.

12. Mrs. R.K. rings her call bell. When you arrive, she has her hand placed over her heart and tells you she is "having that heavy feeling again." She is not diaphoretic or nauseated but states she is short of breath (SOB). What can you do to make her more comfortable.

Note: Laboratory tests can be reported in terms of different values. Always read laboratory reports carefully to be sure which units are used in your institution.

Mrs. R.K.'s husband is very upset. He tells you they have been married for 72 years and he doesn't know what he would do without his wife. One way to help people deal with their anxieties is to help them focus on concrete issues.

13. What information would be useful to get from him? What other health care professional may be able to help with some of these issues?

Case Study 7

Name ______________________ Class/Group ______ Date ______

Group Members ____

INSTRUCTIONS: All questions apply to this case study. Your responses should be brief and to the point. Adequate space has been provided for answers. When asked to provide several answers, they should be listed in order of priority or significance. Do not assume information that is not provided. Please print or write clearly. If your response is not legible, it will be marked as ? and you will need to rewrite it.

Scenario

The time is 1900. You are working in a small, rural hospital. It has been snowing heavily all day, and the medical helicopters at the large regional medical center, 4 hours away by car (in good weather), have been grounded by the weather until morning. The roads are barely passable. W.R., a 48-year-old construction worker with a 36 pack-year smoking history, is admitted to your floor with a diagnosis of R/O MI. He has significant male-pattern obesity ("beer belly," large waist circumference), a barrel chest, and reports a dietary history of high-fat food. His wife brought him to the ED after he complained of unrelieved "indigestion." His admission VS were 202/124, 96, 18, 36.8° C. W.R. was put on O_2/nc titrated to maintain SaO_2 >90% and an IV of NTG was started in the ED. He was also given ASA 325 mg and was admitted to Dr. Adam's service. There are plans to transfer him by chopper to the regional medical center for a cardiac catheterization in the morning when the weather clears. Meanwhile, you have to deal with limited laboratory and pharmacy resources. The minute W.R. comes through the door of your unit, he announces he's just fine in a loud and angry voice and demands a cigarette.

1. From the perspective of basic human needs, what is the first priority in his care?

2. Are these VS reasonable for a man his age? If not, which one(s) concern(s) you. Explain why or why not.

3. Identify five priority problems associated with the care of a patient like W.R.

4. Which of the following laboratory tests might be ordered to investigate W.R.'s condition? If the order is appropriate, place an "A" in the space provided. If inappropriate, mark with an "I."

___ CBC

___ EG in the AM

___ Chem 7 (electrolytes)

___ PT/PTT

___ Bilirubin q AM

___ Urinalysis

___ STAT 12-lead ECG

___ Type and cross (T&C) for 4 units PRCs (packed red cells)

5. What significant laboratory tests are missing from the previous list? ❍ ❍ ❍ ❍ ❍

6. How are you going to respond to W.R.'s angry demands for a cigarette? He also demands something for his "heartburn." How will you respond? ❍ ❍ ❍ ❍ ❍

You phone Dr. Adam's partner who is "on call." She prescribes 10 mg morphine sulfate IV push q1h prn for pain (burning, pressure, angina).

7. Explain two reasons for this order. ❍ ❍ ❍ ❍ ❍

8. What special precautions should you follow when administering morphine sulfate IV push? ❍ ❍ ❍ ❍ ❍

9. Angina is not always experienced as "pain" (as many people understand pain). How would you describe symptoms you want him to warn you about? Why is this important? ❍ ❍ ❍ ❍ ❍

10. What safety measures/instructions would you give W.R. before you leave his room?

11. One of the housekeeping staff asks you, "If the poor guy can't smoke, why can't you give him one of those nicotine patches?" How will you respond?

12. If the patch were to be used later to help him quit smoking, how would it be dosed for him?

HINT: Manufacturers recommend starting with a 14-mg patch for each pack per day the person is smoking.

13. Before leaving for the night, Mrs. R. approaches you and asks, "Did my husband have a heart attack? I'm really scared. His father died of one when he was 51." How are you going to respond to her question?

14. When you come into W.R.'s room at 2200 to answer his call light, you see he is holding his left arm and complaining of (c/o) aching in his left shoulder and arm. What information are you going to gather? What questions will you ask him?

15. Based on your assessment findings, you decide to call the physician. What information are you going to report to her and why?

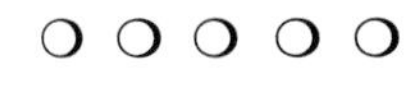

In the morning, W.R. is transferred by chopper to the medical center and a cardiac catheterization is performed. It is determined that W.R. has CAD. The cardiologist suggests it would be best to treat him medically for now with follow-up counseling on risk factor modification, especially smoking cessation. He is discharged with a referral for a follow-up visit to his local internist in 1 week.

16. What does it mean to treat him "medically" (conservatively)? What other approaches may be used to treat coronary artery disease?

17. What personality characteristic do you observe in W.R. that places him at high risk for coronary artery disease?

Case Study 8

Name ______________________ Class/Group ______ Date ______

Group Members ____

INSTRUCTIONS: All questions apply to this case study. Your responses should be brief and to the point. Adequate space has been provided for answers. When asked to provide several answers, they should be listed in order of priority or significance. Do not assume information that is not provided. Please print or write clearly. If your response is not legible, it will be marked as ? and you will need to rewrite it.

Scenario

You are just getting caught up with your work when you receive the following phone call: "Hi, this is Deb in the ED. We're sending you Mrs. M.M., a 63-year-old Hispanic woman with a PMH of CAD. Her daughter reports that she's become increasingly weak over the last couple weeks and has been unable to do her housework. Apparently she has been c/o swelling in her ankles and feet by late afternoon ("she can't wear her shoes") and has nocturnal diuresis x 4. Her daughter brought her in because she has c/o heaviness in her chest off and on over the last few days but denies any discomfort at this time. The daughter took her to see her family physician, who immediately sent her here. VS are 146/92, 96, 24, 37.2° C. She has an IV of D_5W at KVO in her right forearm. Her labs are as follows: Na 134 mmol/L, K 3.5 mmol/L, Cl 103 mmol/L, HCO_3 23, BUN 13 mg/dL, creatinine 1.3 mg/dL, glucose 153 mg/dL, WBC 8.3 thou/cmm, Hct 33.9%, Hgb 11.7 g/dL, platelets 162 thou/cmm. (Note: The former *mm^3* is currently written *Thou* or *thou/cmm.*) PT/INR, PTT, and UA are pending. She has had her CXR and ECG, and her orders have been written."

1. What additional information do you need from the ED nurse?

2. How are you going to prepare for this patient?

3. Name three types of sphygmomonometers.

4. Monitoring her BP is going to be very important. What would you do to check the cuff and tubing to make certain they are in good working order? (List at least three things.)

5. Mrs. M.M. arrives by wheelchair (w/c). As she transfers from the w/c to the bed, what observations should you make? Why?

6. Given the previous information, which of the following orders can you anticipate as appropriate for this patient? Carefully review each order to determine whether it is appropriate or inappropriate as written. If the order is appropriate, place an "A" in the space provided; if the order is inappropriate, place an "I" in the space provided and change the order to make it appropriate. Also provide any other orders that may be appropriate for this patient.

___ Routine VS.

___ Serum magnesium STAT.

___ Up ad lib.

___ 10 g sodium, low animal fat diet.

___ Change IV to normal saline (NS) at 100 ml/h.

___ Cardiac enzymes on admission and q8h x 24 then qAM.

___ CBC (hemogram), Chem 7, and lipid profile in AM.

___ Schedule for abdominal CT scan for AM.

___ Heparin 10,000 U SQ q8h.

___ Docusate sodium 100 mg PO qd.

___ Ampicillin 250 mg IVPB q6h.

___ Furosemide 200 mg IVP STAT.

___ Nitroglycerin 0.4 mg 1 SL q4h prn for chest pain.

7. When you respond to M.M.'s call light, you observe she is talking rapidly in Spanish and pointing to the bathroom. Her speech pattern indicates she is SOB (she is having trouble completing a sentence without taking a labored breath). You assist her to the bathroom and note that her skin feels clammy. While sitting on the commode, she vomits. On a scale of 0 to 10 (0 being no problem, 10 being a CODE-level emergency), how would you rate this situation and why?

8. Identify at least four actions you should take next, and state your rationale.

9. The physician calls your unit to find out what is happening. What information would you need to convey at this time?

10. The resident is coming to the floor to evaluate the patient immediately. In the meantime she orders furosemide 40 mg IVP STAT. You have only 20 mg in stock. Should you give the 20 mg now, then give the additional 20 mg when it comes up from the pharmacy? Explain your answer.

11. M.M. continues to experience vomiting and diaphoresis that are unrelieved by medication and comfort measures. A STAT 12-lead ECG reveals ischemic changes. The patient is transferred to the coronary care unit (CCU). As you give report to the receiving RN, what laboratory value is the most important to report and why?

12. While recovering in ICU, M.M. slipped in the bathroom and fractured her R humerus. Because of the surgical risks involved, M.M. was treated conservatively and put in a full arm cast. She is placed on prophylactic heparin and is again transferred to your floor. A case manager (CM) has been asked to evaluate M.M.'s home to see whether she can be discharged to her own home or will need to stay in a long-term care facility. Identify 8 things that the CM would assess.

13. M.M.'s nutritional intake over the past few weeks has been poor. She also has increased nutritional needs because of her fractured arm. What are some of the nutritional needs that should be met? What would you recommend to help her with this?

Since it is determined that Mrs. M.M. lived in an apartment with poor access, she elects to stay with her daughter and 5 grandchildren in their small home. A home care nurse comes 3 times a week to check on her. M.M. is easily fatigued, and the children are quite lively. School is out for the summer.

14. Suggest some ways the daughter can ensure that her mother isn't overwhelmed and doesn't become exhausted in this situation.

Case Study 9

Name ______________________ Class/Group ______ Date ______

Group Members ______________________________________

INSTRUCTIONS: All questions apply to this case study. Your responses should be brief and to the point. Adequate space has been provided for answers. When asked to provide several answers, they should be listed in order of priority or significance. Do not assume information that is not provided. Please print or write clearly. If your response is not legible, it will be marked as ? and you will need to rewrite it.

Scenario

You are assigned to care for L.J., a 70-year-old retired bus driver who has just been admitted to your medical floor with R leg deep vein thrombosis (DVT). L.J. has a 48 pack-year smoking history, although he states he quit 2 years ago. He has had pneumonia several times and frequent episodes of atrial fibrillation (A fib). He has had 2 previous episodes of DVT and was diagnosed with rheumatoid arthritis 3 years ago. Two months ago he began experiencing SOB on exertion and noticed swelling of his R foreleg that became progressively worse until it also involved his thigh to the groin. His wife brought him to the hospital when he c/o increasingly severe pain in his leg. When a Doppler study indicated a probable thrombus of the external iliac vein extending distally to the lower leg, he was admitted for bed rest and to initiate heparin therapy. Significant admission lab values are PT 12.4 sec, INR 1.11, PTT 25 sec, Hgb 13.3 g/dL, Hct 38.9%, cholesterol 206 mg/dL. Basic metabolic panel is normal.

1. Look up the external iliac vein in your anatomy book. List six risk factors for DVT.

2. Identify at least five problems from L.J.'s history that represent his personal risk factors.

3. Something is missing from the above scenario. Based on his history, L.J. should be taking an important medication. What is it, and why should he be taking it?

4. Keeping in mind L.J.'s health history and admitting diagnosis, what are the most important assessments you should make during your physical examination and assessment?

5. What is the most serious complication of DVT?

Your assessment of L.J. reveals bibasilar crackles with moist cough; normal heart sounds; BP 138/88; P 104; 3+ pitting edema R lower extremity; mild erythema of R foot and calf; and severe R calf pain. He is alert and oriented (AAO) but a little restless. He denies SOB and chest pain.

6. List at least eight assessment findings you should monitor closely for development of the complication identified in question 5.

Note: If a pulmonary embolism is massive, the s/s are more like those of myocardial infarction: crushing, substernal chest pain, marked respiratory distress, feeling of impending doom, rapid, shallow breathing, bloody sputum, severe SOB, dysrhythmias, and shock.

L.J. is placed on 72° BR with BRP and given acetaminophen (Tylenol) for pain.

7. Enoxaparin 70 mg (0.7 ml) is prescribed for systemic anticoagulation. L.J. is 5'6" and weighs 156 lb. What kind of drug is enoxaparin? Is this dose appropriate? How would it be administered?

8. What instructions will you give L.J. about his activity?

Note: Significant others often want to do something helpful. Having them remind the patient to do their ankle exercises, in particular, can be valuable.

9. What pertinent laboratory values/test results would you expect the physician to order and you to monitor?

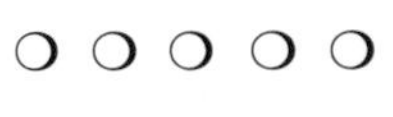

10. You identify pain as a key issue in the care of L.J. List 4 interventions you would choose for L.J. to address his pain.

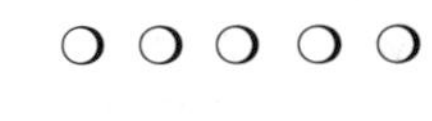

11. (Optional) This is a copy of one of the ECG's taken for L.J. Identify rate; rhythm; QRS after each P; PR interval; and QRS interval. Are sinus and ventricular rhythm the same? Name this rhythm.

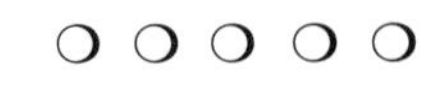

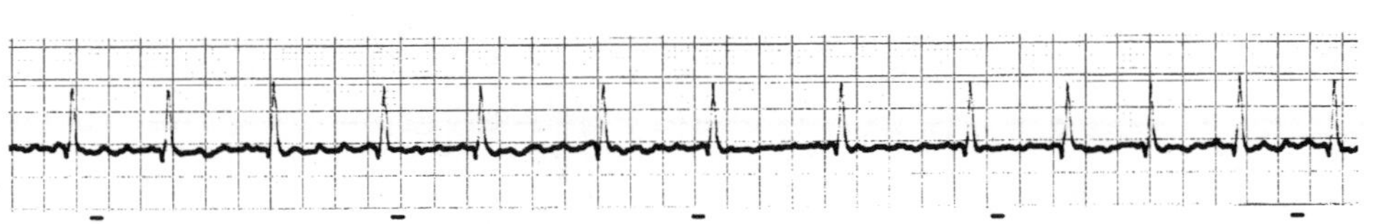

A week has passed. L.J. responded to heparin therapy, was started on warfarin (Coumadin) therapy, and is being discharged to home with home care follow-up. “Good,” he says, “just in time to fly out West for my grandson’s wedding.” His wife, who has come to pick him up, rolls her eyes and looks at the ceiling. You almost drop the discharge papers in disbelief at what you have just heard. (And you thought you did such a good job of discharge teaching!)

12. What are you going to tell him?

L.J. listens to you, and Mrs. J. is quite relieved. (She has been telling her friends about this “wonderful nurse who talked some sense into my husband.”) L.J.’s son arranges to videotape the entire wedding ceremony, and guests at the reception tape special greetings for him. It’s been 2 weeks, and he seems quite pleased. He watches the tape daily and points out his favorite parts to the home care nurse every time she visits.

Case Study 10

Name ______________________ Class/Group ______ Date ______

Group Members ______________________________

INSTRUCTIONS: All questions apply to this case study. Your responses should be brief and to the point. Adequate space has been provided for answers. When asked to provide several answers, they should be listed in order of priority or significance. Do not assume information that is not provided. Please print or write clearly. If your response is not legible, it will be marked as ? and you will need to rewrite it.

❍ ❍ ❍ / ❍ ❍

Scenario

J.T. is a 58-year-old Tongan man admitted to your floor with syncope and right-sided heart failure. He was brought to the hospital after "passing out" and "turning blue" for 2 minutes after a severe bout of coughing. Because J.T. speaks very little English, his wife helps you obtain his health history: type 2 DM, significant abdominal obesity, hypertension, CHF, chronic hypoxia, frequent pneumonia, hyperlipidemia, and polycythemia. His wife tells you he snores loudly and seems to stop breathing sometimes during the night. He has no history of smoking or alcohol use. His weight is 360 pounds. Over the last week he has had intermittent chest pain with SOB on exertion. The SOB has increased during the last 12 hours. He has been hospitalized in the past for chest pain but has never been diagnosed with an MI. On admission today he has orthopnea, a severe dry cough, palpitations, and SOB. He is not c/o chest pain or discomfort. His VS are 166/104, 94, 22, 36.7° C. You hear muffled S_1 and S_2 heart sounds and a possible S_3. He has moderate pretibial edema to his knees and a few bibasilar crackles. You place him on oxygen at 3 L/min by nasal cannula and insert a Foley catheter. His blood glucose level is 347 mg/dL and Hct is 50%. Cholesterol and triglyceride levels are 320 mg/dL and 266 mg/dL, respectively.

1. What is the relationship of J.T.'s country of origin to his current health problems? ❍ ❍ ❍ ❍ ❍

2. From the scenario presented, J.T. has hyperglycemia, hypertension, and hyperlipidemia. What is the evidence for each? In what order should they be addressed, and why? ❍ ❍ ❍ ❍ ❍

3. What do you think is the significance of J.T.'s wife's report about his snoring and sleep-related breathing pattern?

4. Judging from the admission information, do you think he has right-sided CHF, left-sided CHF, or both? Cite your evidence.

5. List three other things you could assess to confirm your suspicion of right-sided heart failure.

6. What class of medication could be used to treat his CHF and hypertension and to prevent diabetic nephropathy? What beneficial actions of these medications, in particular, would help J.T.?

7. What is a possible explanation for his chronic hypoxia?

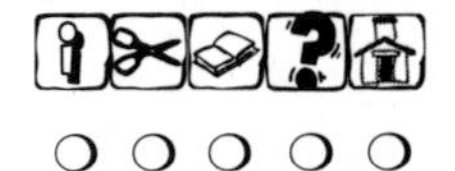

8. List four priority nursing problems r/t J.T.'s care. ❍ ❍ ❍ ❍ ❍

The night shift nurse confirms the report that J.T. snores loudly ("I could hear him all the way down the hall!") and "has 30- to 60-second pauses in his breathing followed by a violent jerk and thrashing as he resumes inspirations." A sleep study is ordered.

9. Define a sleep study, and explain what information can be obtained from it. ❍ ❍ ❍ ❍ ❍

The sleep study shows obstructive sleep apnea with oxygen desaturation as low as 32% for prolonged periods following each apneic episode. During his study, J.T. had over 320 apneic episodes in 1 night.

10. Continuous positive airway pressure (CPAP) is prescribed for J.T. Explain the concept of CPAP and how it will benefit him. ❍ ❍ ❍ ❍ ❍

On the second day after admission, J.T. developed chills and fever with a temperature of 38.5° C and an SaO_2 of 88% on 3L O_2/nc. The physician suggests he is developing an infection.

11. What are the two most likely sources of infection that might be responsible for J.T.'s fever? ❍ ❍ ❍ ❍ ❍

While waiting for the results of the C&S, the physician starts J.T. on azithromycin and cefuroxime (broad-spectrum ATB) for bacterial pneumonitis. During his hospitalization, J.T.'s family has been bringing him food and drinks from home despite explanations by the nurses that he is on a 2000-calorie, low-salt, diabetic diet, and he is on fluid restriction. Because of his obesity and extreme SOB on exertion, he is quite immobilized.

12. When and how should his antibiotics be administered? What laboratory tests should be monitored for complications?

13. Identify the most serious complication of immobility for which J.T. is at risk, and state the reasons for this risk. What prophylactic intervention would be used to address this risk?

After a week on ATB for his pneumonitis and diuresis for his CHF, J.T.'s doctor says he is ready to go home. You have developed a list of things that you think he and his family should be taught before he is ready for discharge. After reviewing his history, you have decided that he has many risk factors for CAD; although he has not had an MI yet, he is at risk for having one. You have placed teaching about cardiac risk factors at the top of your list.

14. List 4 cardiac risk factors that J. T. has and place a check mark beside the ones that are potentially modifiable through behavioral change.

15. Identify two major pathologic conditions J.T. has for which he needs teaching. ❍ ❍ ❍ ❍ ❍

16. What do you think is the likelihood J.T. will be motivated to exercise and diet to lose weight, and why? ❍ ❍ ❍ ❍ ❍

At the recommendation of the case manager, the HMO has secured the services of an RD who served a mission to Tonga with the Church of Jesus Christ of Latter Day Saints. She speaks the language and understands the culture. She will work with J.T.'s family to address dietary issues, focusing on the dietary aspects of managing his type 2 DM, CHF, and hyperlipidemia—within his cultural context.

Case Study 11

Name ______________________ Class/Group ______ Date ______

Group Members ______________________

INSTRUCTIONS: All questions apply to this case study. Your responses should be brief and to the point. Adequate space has been provided for answers. When asked to provide several answers, they should be listed in order of priority or significance. Do not assume information that is not provided. Please print or write clearly. If your response is not legible, it will be marked as ? and you will need to rewrite it.

Scenario

L.M. is a 60-year-old woman who is admitted to your telemetry unit in a major medical center after being successfully resuscitated by medics from a cardiac arrest due to ventricular fibrillation (V fib). L.M., a divorced housewife, had her sudden death experience in the small rural community where she lives and was transported to your facility for evaluation and treatment after she was stabilized. At the time of the arrest, her K level was 2.8 mmol/L and Mg level was 1.3 mg/dL. As you continue to review her medical history, you learn that she had rheumatic fever as a child and over the years has developed severe rheumatic heart disease with mitral and aortic valve involvement and dilated cardiomyopathy. Four years ago she had a commissurotomy for mitral valve stenosis. She also has probable aortic valve stenosis. During the past year she has experienced increasing problems with chest pain, SOB, and dyspnea on exertion. Two months ago she developed a severe cough and increasing fatigue. She has been on furosemide 40 mg PO qd, digoxin 0.125 mg PO qd, captopril 50 mg PO q8h, and potassium (K Dur) 20 mEq PO qd. In addition, during the week before her cardiac arrest, she was taking erythromycin 500 mg PO q6h for a lower respiratory tract infection. Although she stopped smoking 4 years ago, she had a 40 pack-year smoking history.

1. What organism causes rheumatic fever?

2. What is a mitral valve commissurotomy, and how is it carried out?

3. What medication is commonly used prophylactically to prevent development of rheumatic heart disease when an individual has rheumatic fever?

4. Why would someone like L.M. be given Coumadin?

5. Reviewing the above health history, what factors do you think contribute to her current symptoms of chest pain, SOB, dyspnea on exertion, cough, and fatigue? Explain your rationale for each.

6. What factors in the above health history may have precipitated L.M.'s cardiac arrest?

L.M.'s admission VS are 102/60, 84, 16, and 36° C. Her telemetry monitor shows A fib and frequent PVCs. When you listen to her heart, you hear an S_3 gallop, a grade III/VI systolic murmur, and a soft, blowing diastolic murmur. Her PMI is displaced laterally. She has no pedal edema. You hear crackles in her lungs. Other assessment findings are normal. She is transferred to the CCU and is placed on continuous heparin and lidocaine IV infusions, and started on O_2 at 40% by face mask. Her lab values are drawn. Later in the day during a cardiac catheterization, her cardiac output (CO) was found to be 2.3 L/min and her mean pulmonary artery pressure 29 mm Hg.

7. Based on the above assessment, do you believe that L.M. is experiencing some heart failure? Why or why not?

8. L.M.'s lab tests return. Her PT is 23.4 seconds/INR = 1.99, PTT 30 seconds. What other lab tests would you especially want to monitor?

9. Why is it important to monitor L.M.'s PTT? Is her PTT within the therapeutic range? Is the PT within the normal range? ❍ ❍ ❍ ❍ ❍

10. What would be the advantages and disadvantages of giving L.M. Pen VK versus erythromycin (list at least one in each category)? ❍ ❍ ❍ ❍ ❍

11. List four relevant problems r/t L.M.'s nursing care. ❍ ❍ ❍ ❍ ❍

12. In order to prevent serious complications, you will assess and monitor for potential problems. List three significant potential physiologic problems for which L.M. is at risk. Explain.

13. The technologic monitoring and care L.M. receives demands so much time that there has been little opportunity to talk with her about her feelings r/t her sudden death experience. As you plan to approach her, you remind yourself to be sensitive to communication limitations imposed by her pathologic condition. What are two of these limitations, and how will they affect your interaction?

Case Study 12

Name ______________________ Class/Group ______ Date ______

Group Members ______________________________________

INSTRUCTIONS: All questions apply to this case study. Your responses should be brief and to the point. Adequate space has been provided for answers. When asked to provide several answers, they should be listed in order of priority or significance. Do not assume information that is not provided. Please print or write clearly. If your response is not legible, it will be marked as ? and you will need to rewrite it.

❍ ❍ ❍ / ❍ ❍

Scenario

T.G. is a 34-year-old woman who was admitted to your CCU with an anterior wall MI secondary to cocaine use. Upon arrival in the unit, she still has the nitroglycerine (NTG) drip infusing that had been started in the ambulance and maintained in the ED. You are instructed to titrate the drip for relief of her chest pain. Her maintenance IV is D_5½NS at 100 mL/h. O_2 per n/c (N/C) is to be titrated to keep her SaO_2 >90%. As you assess T.G., she reports relief of her chest and L arm pain but says that a dull chest pressure persists; she denies tenderness with light pressure to her chest. Her cardiovascular and pulmonary assessments are otherwise normal. She has a headache and is drowsy, but aware of her surroundings and oriented. ED VS were 136/97, 79, 20, 37.2° C. Her weight is listed as 92 pounds; height 5'2".

The report from the ED nurse is as follows: "T.G. is a single woman with 3 children; she works as a clerk in a small chain grocery store. The family is on Medicaid; they live with her boyfriend. We're also betting she's been 'hooking' on the side for drug money, but she refused to discuss it. She has smoked 1½ packs of cigarettes a day for 20 years and has chronic hepatitis B. Although she is evasive about her street drug use, medical records from a prior admission suggest she also has an 18-year history of cocaine and IV heroin addiction. When using heroin, she admits to injecting the drug 2 to 3 times per day. There are no visible track marks on her arms or legs, but it looks like she's been shooting up between her toes and in her breasts. Last night she administered the cocaine by intravenous injection for the first time in an attempt to 'stop the heroin habit.' She felt all right when she went to bed just before midnight, but woke about 0500 with severe chest pain radiating to her L arm and hand, neck, and both sides of her jaw. She also had N/V, SOB, diaphoresis, and dizziness. Her boyfriend called 911, and she was brought here by ambulance. She reports pain rated as 9/10."

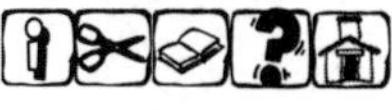
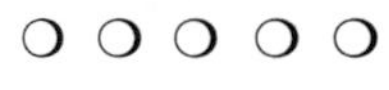

1. The ED nurse told you T.G. reported pain as 9/10, but she tells you her chest pain is relieved. List two possible reasons to account for the discrepancy.

2. What nursing problems would you identify for T.G.? List your four top-priority problems, and give the evidence for each.

You look up the effects of cocaine and find that the 2 primary acute effects on the cardiovascular system are (1) blocking of the reuptake of catecholamines, resulting in increased stimulation of both alpha-adrenergic receptors (vasoconstriction) and beta-adrenergic receptors (increased heart rate and increased cardiac automaticity); and (2) blocking of the fast-sodium channel in the myocardium, resulting in depression of depolarization and a slowing of conduction velocity (local anesthetic effect). In addition, myocardial contractility is suppressed. Chronic cocaine leads to acceleration of atherosclerosis and increased tendency for platelet aggregation.

3. Based on this information, what possible ECG changes due to cocaine toxicity would you monitor for?

4. What physiologic complications of cocaine toxicity would you monitor for? Identify three.

5. Review the previous data on the effects of cocaine. List ways by which cocaine use may lead to myocardial infarction.

6. What laboratory test may give the best general indication of T.G.'s nutritional status?

7. In view of T.G.'s suspected sexual behavior history, what other laboratory tests would you anticipate?

8. The day after she is admitted, T.G. begins to appear anxious, depressed, restless, and irritable. She is doubled over and c/o abdominal cramping. You also notice muscle twitching and tremors. She refuses to eat, saying she feels nauseated. To what do you attribute these symptoms?

9. In response to your call, the physician ordered methadone 10 mg PO tid for T.G. What is the rationale for prescribing methadone in this instance?

10. Before T.G. is transferred to the step-down telemetry floor, you consult with the social worker to identify her discharge needs. List at least two.

11. What danger is associated with her taking methadone?

Shortly after T.G. is moved to the telemetry unit, her telemetry alarm sounds. When you go into her room, you find her disconnected telemetry unit and leads on her bed, and she is nowhere to be found. Her $D_5 \frac{1}{2}$NS IV has been pulled out and is dripping into the bed. When she returns about an hour later, she is very mellow and easy-going, almost lethargic. She immediately falls asleep and is difficult to arouse.

12. To what do you attribute her absence and her present behavior?

Note: Nearly every large hospital in the country is covered by one or more drug dealers. Hospital personnel and patients who are abusing drugs need their "fix" or "hit" and are willing to pay well for it. Drug dealers are willing to oblige with personalized service.

13. What is going to be your response to the above situation?

14. What drug may be administered to reverse the effects of a narcotic overdose? What risks could it impose in a situation like this?

15. As you take her pulse, you notice that her respirations are now 6 per minute and shallow. Her pulse is irregular, and you cannot rouse her. What are you going to do?

16. (Optional) The telemetry alarm sounds. On the screen above her bed, you see the rhythm strip image shown in "A" below. What has happened, and what is the significance?

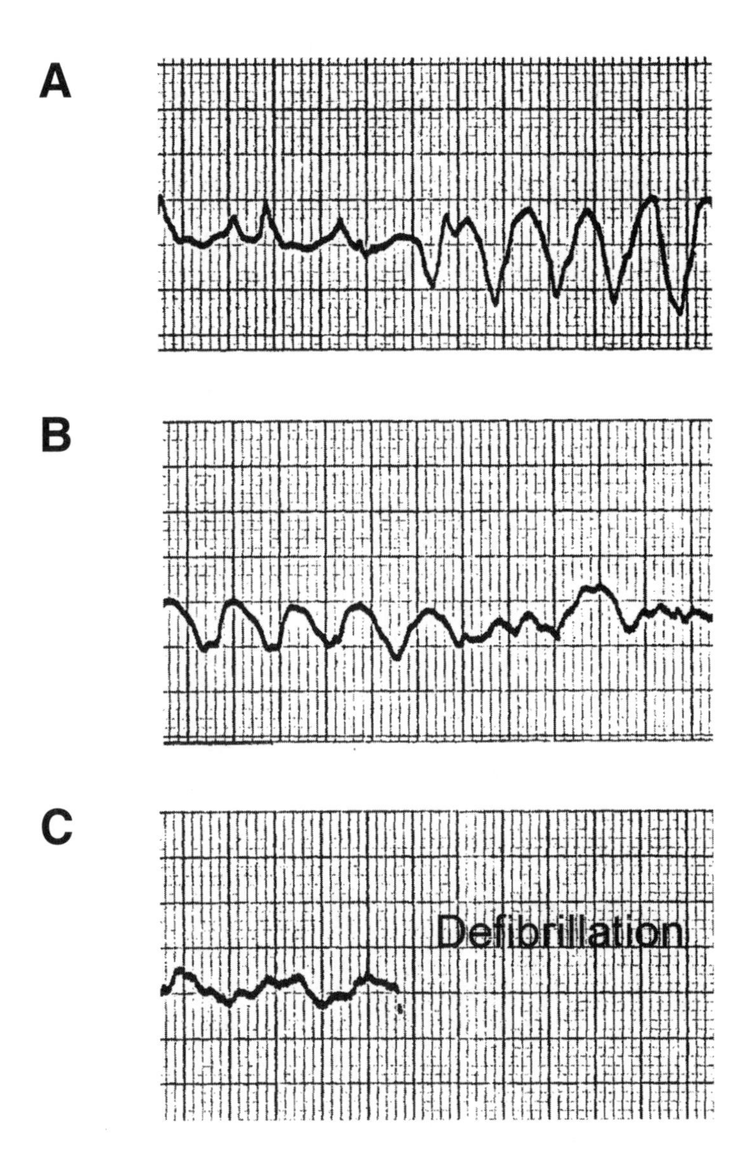

Within seconds, the pattern changes (B) from V tach to V fib. Your support team arrives and the defibrillator is charged up. "Everybody off!" C shows the temporary pattern disruption produced by the electrical discharge. When the pattern stabilizes, she is still in V fib. Although the team works on T.G. for nearly 30 minutes, they are unable to establish a stable cardiac rhythm. She is declared dead, and you are left to clean up after her and after the code. To see the protocol (like a recipe) for Advanced Cardiac Life Support (ACLS) that would be used by the team in a setting like this, look it up at the American Heart Association's Web site. Other Web sites have excellent "code" simulations as well. As a student, if you have a patient who "codes," you must be aware of the patient's DNR (do not resuscitate) status. If they are to be resuscitated, call for help, start CPR, and then get out of the way when help comes.

Case Study 13

Name ______________________ Class/Group ______ Date ______

Group Members ______________________________________

INSTRUCTIONS: All questions apply to this case study. Your responses should be brief and to the point. Adequate space has been provided for answers. When asked to provide several answers, they should be listed in order of priority or significance. Do not assume information that is not provided. Please print or write clearly. If your response is not legible, it will be marked as ? and you will need to rewrite it.

Scenario

You are working in the internal medicine clinic of a large teaching hospital. Today your first patient is 70-year-old J.M., a man who has been coming to the clinic for several years for management of CAD, hypertension, and anemia. A cardiac catheterization done a year ago showed 50% occlusion of the circumflex coronary artery. He has had episodes of dizziness for the past 6 months and orthostatic hypotension, shoulder discomfort, and decreased exercise tolerance for the past 2 months. On his last clinic visit 3 weeks ago, a CXR and 12-lead ECG were done, showing cardiomegaly and an LBBB. Results of chemistries (blood studies) drawn at this time were as follows: Na 136 mmol/L, K 5.2 mmol/L, BUN 15 mg/dL, creatinine 1.8 mg/dL, glucose 82 mg/dL, Cl 95 mmol/L, CBC: WBC 4.4 thou/cmm, Hgb 10.5 g/dL, Hct 31.4%, and platelets 229 thou/cmm. This morning his daughter has brought him to the clinic because he has had increased fatigue, significant swelling of his ankles, and SOB for the last 2 days. His VS are 142/83, 105, 18, and 36.6° C.

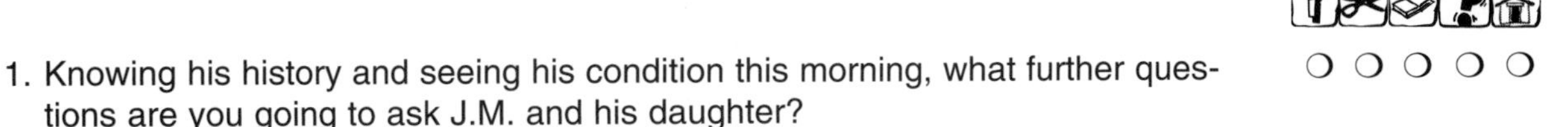

1. Knowing his history and seeing his condition this morning, what further questions are you going to ask J.M. and his daughter?

J.M. tells you he becomes exhausted and SOB climbing the stairs to his bedroom and has to lie down and rest ("put my feet up") at least an hour twice a day. He has been sleeping on 2 pillows for the last 2 weeks. He has not salted his food since the doctor told him not to because of his high BP. But he admits having had ham and a whole bag of salted peanuts 3 days ago. He denies having palpitations but has had a constant, irritating, nonproductive cough lately.

2. You think it likely that J.M. has congestive heart failure. From his history, what do you identify as probable causes for his CHF?

3. You are now ready to do your physical assessment. List at least nine things you would assess to confirm your suspicion about the CHF. Also indicate with an "L" or an "R" whether the sign is due to left-sided or right-sided heart failure or both.

4. The doctor confirms your feelings that J.M. is experiencing some CHF. What classes of medications might the doctor prescribe? ❍ ❍ ❍ ❍ ❍

Note: The Hgb and Hct might be falsely decreased because of hemodilution of the CHF.

5. This is J.M.'s first episode of significant CHF. Before he leaves the clinic, you want to teach him about lifestyle modifications he can make and monitoring techniques he can use to prevent or minimize future problems. List five suggestions you might make and the rationale for each. ❍ ❍ ❍ ❍ ❍

6. You tell J.M. the combination of sodium-high foods he had during the past several days may have set off his present episode of CHF. He looks surprised. J.M. says, "But I didn't add any salt to them!" To what health care professional could he be referred to help him understand how to prevent future crises? State your rationale. ❍ ❍ ❍ ❍ ❍

7. J.M. receives a prescription for furosemide with a potassium supplement. He wrinkles his nose at the suggestion of potassium and tells you he "hates those horse pills." He tells you a friend of his said he could eat bananas, instead. He says he would rather eat a banana every day than take one of those pills. How will you respond?

8. It's winter and today's temperature is 15° F. J.M. tells you he's been getting cold feet lately. This has never bothered him before. What would you suggest as comfort and safety measures?

9. Researchers sometimes call the legs "the second heart." In view of this statement and J.M.'s cardiac history, explain why "walking would be better than standing" for his circulation.

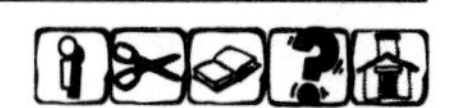

J.M.'s daughter is interested in knowing how she can read the nutritional information on food labels so that she can be a wiser shopper when she gets his groceries.

10. Using the food labels below, provide a plain-English explanation of what the various pieces of information mean. Especially discuss the sodium content in "A" (skim milk) versus the sodium content in "B" (boxed macaroni and cheese). ❍ ❍ ❍ ❍ ❍

A

Nutrition Facts
Serving Size 1 cup (240 mL)
Servings Per Container About 16

Amount Per Serving	
Calories 80 Calories from Fat 0	
	% **Daily Value***
Total Fat 0g	**0%**
Saturated fat 0g	**0%**
Cholesterol Less than 5mg	**1%**
Sodium 125mg	**5%**
Total Carbohydrate 13g	**4%**
Dietary Fiber 0g	**0%**
Sugars 13g	
Protein 8g	
Vitamin A 10% Vitamin C 4%	
Calories 30% Iron 0% Vitamin D 25%	

* Percent Daily Values are based on a 2000 calorie diet. Your daily values may be higher or lower depending on your calorie needs.

B

Nutrition Facts
Serving Size 2.5 oz. (1 cup prepared)
(68g about 1/2 cup dry macaroni and 4 tsp dry cheese mix)
Servings Per Container 3

Amount Per Serving	**In Package**	**As Prepared**
Calories	250	390
Calories from Fat	15	140
	% **Daily Value***	
Total Fat 1.5g	**2%**	**25%**
Saturated Fat 0.5g	**2%**	**25%**
Cholesterol less than 5mg	**0%**	**0%**
Sodium 640mg	**26%**	**32%**
Total Carbohydrates 50g	**17%**	**17%**
Dietary Fiber 2g	**8%**	**8%**
Sugars 5g		
Protein 8g		

* Percent Daily Values are based on a 2000 calorie diet. Your daily values may be higher or lower depending on your calorie needs.

Case Study 14

Name ______________________ Class/Group ______ Date ______

Group Members ____

INSTRUCTIONS: All questions apply to this case study. Your responses should be brief and to the point. Adequate space has been provided for answers. When asked to provide several answers, they should be listed in order of priority or significance. Do not assume information that is not provided. Please print or write clearly. If your response is not legible, it will be marked as ? and you will need to rewrite it.

❍ ❍ ❍ / ❍ ❍

Scenario

J.M. is a 70-year-old retired construction worker who has experienced lumbosacral pain, nausea, and upset stomach for the past 6 months. He has a history of CHF, deep visceral pain, dyspnea, hypertension, and depression. J.M. has just been admitted to the hospital for surgical repair of a 6.2-cm abdominal aortic aneurysm (AAA), which is now causing him constant pain. Upon arrival on your floor, his VS are 109/81, 61, 16 and 98.3° F. When you perform your assessment, you find that his apical heart rhythm is regular and his peripheral pulses are strong. His lungs are clear, and he is AAO. There are no abnormal physical findings; however, he hasn't had a bowel movement for 3 days. His electrolytes and other blood chemistries and clotting studies are within normal range, but his Hct is 30.1% and Hgb 9.0 g/dL.

J.M. has been depressed since the death of his wife 9 years ago. He has no children. His height is 6'2" and weight 160 lb. His chronic medical problems have been managed over the years by medications: benazepril 40 mg PO qd, fluoxetine 40 mg PO qd, furosemide 40 mg PO qd, trazodone 50 mg PO qhs, KCl 20 mEq PO bid, and lovastatin 40 mg PO qhs.

❍ ❍ ❍ ❍ ❍

1. J.M. has several common risk factors for AAA, which are evident from his health history. Identify and explain three factors.

While J.M. awaits his surgery, it is important that you monitor him carefully for decrease in tissue perfusion.

2. Identify five things you would assess for, and state your rationale for each.

3. What is the most serious, life-threatening complication of AAA, and why?

4. What single problem mentioned in the first paragraph of this case study presents a risk for AAA rupture? Why?

Monitoring urinary output is critical in evaluating shock or for post-survival problems.

5. What is the minimal acceptable urinary output per hour?

The resection of J.M.'s aneurysm was successful, but for the first 3 postop days he was delirious and required one-to-one nursing care and soft restraints before he became coherent and oriented again. He was still somewhat confused when he was transferred back to your floor.

6. What nursing assessments should be made specific to his aneurysm?

7. List five nursing problems that should be high priorities in J.M.'s postoperative care.

8. Postoperative care of the patient undergoing aneurysectomy includes preservation of the graft, preservation of tissue perfusion, and prevention of infection. List three nursing interventions that would address these issues and explain each.

When J.M. is being prepared for discharge, you talk to him about health promotion and lifestyle change issues that are pertinent to his health problems.

9. Identify four health-related issues you might appropriately address with him and what you would teach in each area.

10. J.M. will be receiving follow-up visits from the home health care nurse to change his dressing and evaluate his incision. What can you discuss with J.M. before discharge that will help him understand what the nurse will be doing?

11. What link could there be between J.M.'s diet and his depression?

Make sure there is a physician's order for medical nutrition therapy for J.M. He is going to need a lot of help with maintaining a healthy diet specific to his needs. RDs are often aware of community resources that could help someone like J.M.

Case Study 15

Name ______________________ Class/Group ______ Date ______

Group Members ______________________________

INSTRUCTIONS: All questions apply to this case study. Your responses should be brief and to the point. Adequate space has been provided for answers. When asked to provide several answers, they should be listed in order of priority or significance. Do not assume information that is not provided. Please print or write clearly. If your response is not legible, it will be marked as ? and you will need to rewrite it.

Scenario

J.C., a 40-year-old married college professor, has just been admitted to your telemetry floor with a diagnosis of "benign ventricular ectopy." He suddenly began experiencing frequent episodes of palpitations 2 years ago. These were accompanied by lightheadedness, weakness, dizziness, and decreased ability to concentrate. Holter monitoring revealed very frequent PVCs exacerbated by caffeine and exertion. On admission, he appears trim, muscular, and physically fit. As you are assessing him, he tells you that he played football in college and has lived a very active lifestyle ever since. He confides that his symptoms seriously interfere with his activities and his marital relationship and cause him a lot of anxiety and depression, to the point where he almost "took his life" a year ago. He has been taking clonazepam for his anxiety for about 18 months. His physician tried 4 different beta-blockers and the antidysrhythmic drug mexiletine to control his PVCs, but none was successful and all had unpleasant side effects. In desperation, J.C. has agreed to try another antidysrhythmic, flecainide, and was admitted for cardiac monitoring. His physical assessment, laboratory values, and cardiac catheterization were normal in all areas.

1. Identify at least two relevant challenges in J.C.'s nursing care.

2. Of the above problems, which is the most potentially life-threatening?

3. When a person is threatened with his or her heart stopping without notice, there is an understandably intense feeling of loss of control and panic. The first objective should be to restore some sense of control to J.C. What are five things you could do to help relieve some of his anxiety?

4. Review each of the following admit orders. If the order is appropriate, place an "A" in the space provided. If it is inappropriate, mark with an "I"; then specify why it is inappropriate, and correct it.

___ Continuous telemetry monitoring.

___ Routine VS.

___ Activity ad lib.

___ Troponin level on admission and CK with isoenzymes q8h x 3.

___ NTG 1 0.4 mg SL prn chest pain.

___ Call physician for PVCs >6/min.

___ Low-cholesterol diet.

___ IV lock.

___ Caffeine restriction.

___ Complete metabolic panel, CBC with differential in AM.

___ 12-lead ECG q AM.

___ Furosemide 40 mg PO qd.

___ Monitor flecainide level as appropriate.

5. List three appropriate nursing interventions r/t J.C.'s dysrhythmia. ❍ ❍ ❍ ❍ ❍

J.C. has just returned to his room from an exercise session in the cardiac rehab room when he collapses on the floor. You witness his fall.

6. What are the appropriate emergency actions you should take? ❍ ❍ ❍ ❍ ❍

According to the cardiac monitor, J.C.'s collapse was due to a sudden episode of V fib. Thanks to a quick response by the hospital's code team, he was successfully defibrillated and resuscitated, then transferred to the CCU.

7. What important information would you include in your report to the CCU nurse who will be caring for J.C.? ❍ ❍ ❍ ❍ ❍

You approach J.C. saying "I think we should notify your wife about your condition." J.C. tells you she is out-of-town on a business trip but calls in regularly for messages. He asks you to call her. Note that if he were unconscious or cognitively impaired, you must notify her since she is the next of kin.

8. J.C.'s wife receives the CCU nurse's message on her answering machine to call the unit. When she returns the call, what information should the nurse tell her? ❍ ❍ ❍ ❍ ❍

She hisses into the telephone, "What the heck do you expect me to do about it. There's no way I'm going to drop a good business deal to run home and hold his hand. He's sure got you fooled. There's nothing wrong with him that a good psychiatrist couldn't fix."

9. As the nurse, how should you respond? ❍ ❍ ❍ ❍ ❍

10. After J.C.'s condition has stabilized, he is referred to the cardiac rehabilitation and prevention program for an exercise prescription. A clinical exercise physiologist helps him develop individualized guidelines for safe exercise. Identify and explain the major components of an exercise prescription.

11. J.C. is used to a much more "macho" approach to exercise: "No pain, no gain." What would be the advantage to him in following an individualized plan drawn up by the exercise physiologist?

The flecainide does not work for J.C. He suffers 3 more significant episodes of V fib over the next 2 months and has to be defibrillated. It is decided that he will receive an implantable cardioverter defibrillator (ICD) or automatic ICD (AICD) to augment the antidysrhythmic drug therapy.

Note: An excellent source of the latest information on the ICD is through the American Heart Association's Web site: *http://www.americanheart.org* under "implantable cardioverter/defibrillator."

12. Briefly describe what an ICD is and how it works. ❍ ❍ ❍ ❍ ❍

13. Does implanting an ICD require open chest surgery? Explain. ❍ ❍ ❍ ❍ ❍

14. List at least three conditions that may cause a ventricular arrhythmia and have to be R/O before an ICD is implanted. ❍ ❍ ❍ ❍ ❍

15. What is one other condition that would be a relative contraindication to ICD therapy? ❍ ❍ ❍ ❍ ❍

Case Study 16

Name ____________________ Class/Group ______ Date ______

Group Members ________________________________

INSTRUCTIONS: All questions apply to this case study. Your responses should be brief and to the point. Adequate space has been provided for answers. When asked to provide several answers, they should be listed in order of priority or significance. Do not assume information that is not provided. Please print or write clearly. If your response is not legible, it will be marked as ? and you will need to rewrite it.

Scenario

Your patient, 58-year-old K.Z., has a significant cardiac history. He has long-standing CAD with occasional episodes of CHF. One year ago he had an anterior wall MI. In addition, he has chronic anemia, hypertension, chronic renal insufficiency, and a recently diagnosed 4-cm suprarenal AAA. Because of his severe CAD, he had to retire from his job as a railroad engineer about 6 months ago. This morning he is being admitted to your telemetry unit for a same-day cardiac catheterization. As you take his health history, you note that his wife died a year ago (about the same time that he had his MI) and that he does not have any children. He is a current cigarette smoker with a 50-pack-year smoking history. As you talk with him, you realize that he has only minimal understanding of the catheterization procedure. His VS are 158/94, 88, 20 and 36.2° C.

1. Before he leaves for the cath lab, you briefly teach him the important things he needs to know before having the procedure. List five priority topics you will address.

Several hours later, K.Z. returns from his catheterization. The cath report shows 90% occlusion of the proximal left anterior descending coronary artery (LAD), 90% occlusion of the distal LAD, 70% to 80% occlusion of the distal right coronary artery (RCA), an old apical infarct, and an ejection fraction of 37%. About an hour after the procedure is finished, you perform a brief physical assessment and find that he now has a carotid bruit, a grade III/VI systolic ejection murmur at the cardiac apex, crackles bilaterally in the lung bases, and trace pitting edema of his feet and ankles. Except for a soft systolic murmur, these findings were not present before the catheterization.

2. Review the location of these vessels on a diagram of the heart from your anatomy book. Sketch (don't trace) a simple illustration of the anterior heart; label the superior and interior vena cava, the pulmonary artery and vein, and the aorta. Draw the main coronary arteries on the surface of the heart. Circle the areas of the LAD and RCA that have significant occlusion. Lightly shade the part of the heart where K.Z. had an earlier infarct. Using the illustration as a patient teaching aid, explain, in plain English, how you would teach him what "37% ejection fraction" means and how you would expect it to influence his everyday activity.

3. What is your evaluation of the catheterization results?

4. What problem do the changes in assessment findings suggest to you? What led you to your conclusion?

Note: Patients usually express statements like, "Something is wrong . . . I just don't feel right." The nurse needs to be alert to this and reassure them that she is listening to them and monitoring their status. Such statements should never be taken lightly. They should be shared with nurses on the next shift and the patient's physician. If you have a chance, discuss this with your instructor and the rest of the class.

5. List four actions you would take as a result of your evaluation of the assessment and state your rationales.

After assessing him, K.Z.'s doctor admits him (with a diagnosis of CAD and CHF) for coronary artery bypass graft (CABG) surgery. Significant lab results drawn at this time are Hct 25.3%, Hgb 8.8 g/dL, BUN 33 mg/dL, and creatinine 3.1 mg/dL. K.Z. is diuresed with furosemide and given 2 units of packed red blood cells (PRCs).

6. Review K.Z.'s health history. Can you identify a probable explanation for his chronic renal insufficiency and anemia?

Five days later, after his condition is stabilized, K.Z. is taken to surgery for bypass of 3 coronary arteries (CABG x 3). When he arrives in the SICU, he has a Swan-Ganz catheter in place for hemodynamic monitoring and is intubated and put on a ventilator at FiO_2 .70 and PEEP 5 cm H_2O. His first hemodynamic readings are as follows: pulmonary artery pressure (PAP) 41/23 mm Hg, CVP 13 mm Hg, PCWP 13 mm Hg, cardiac index (CI) 1.88 L/min/m^2. ABGs drawn at this time are pH 7.36, PCO_2 46 mm Hg, PO_2 61 mm Hg, and SaO_2 85%, with a Hgb 10.3 mg/dL.

7. Why are ABGs necesssary in the case of K.Z.? List two reasons why it would be inappropriate to use pulse oximetry on K.Z. to assess his oxygen saturation status.

8. What is your evaluation of K.Z.'s hemodynamic status based on the previous parameters?

Clinically, these values show that the pressures within his heart and lungs are a little high and that his cardiac output is a little low, indicating that his heart is still having difficulty pumping out all the blood that is returned to it and/or that he is a little fluid overloaded. His condition will require careful monitoring.

9. K.Z. is receiving continuous IV infusions of nitroprusside and dobutamine. He also has just received 2 units of fresh frozen plasma (FFP). Given this information, do you think the hemodynamic values reported above reflect poor L ventricular function or fluid overload and why?

10. Why is K.Z. receiving the nitroprusside and dobutamine?

11. What is your responsibility when administering nitroprusside and dobutamine to your patient?

12. Why did he receive the FFP?

13. Is it possible for K.Z. to experience a transfusion reaction when receiving albumin or FFP infusion? Explain your answer.

14. What is your interpretation of his ABGs on 70% O_2?

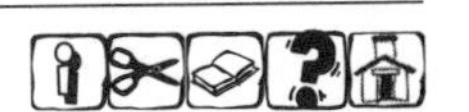

After 3 days in the SICU, K.Z.'s condition is stable and he is returned to your telemetry floor. Now, 5 days later, he is ready to go home, and you are preparing him for discharge.

15. List at least two specific areas of teaching that he should receive r/t his cardiac catheterization.

16. List at least four general areas r/t his CABG surgery in which he should receive instruction before he goes home.

Case Study 17

Name ____________________ Class/Group ______ Date ______

Group Members ______________________________

INSTRUCTIONS: All questions apply to this case study. Your responses should be brief and to the point. Adequate space has been provided for answers. When asked to provide several answers, they should be listed in order of priority or significance. Do not assume information that is not provided. Please print or write clearly. If your response is not legible, it will be marked as ? and you will need to rewrite it.

Scenario

C.W., a 70-year-old man, was brought to the ED at 0430 this morning by his wife. She told the ED triage nurse that he had dysentery for the past 3 days and last night he had a lot of "dark red" diarrhea. When he became very dizzy, disoriented, and weak this morning, she decided to bring him to the hospital. C.W.'s VS were systolic BP 70 mm Hg, diastolic BP inaudible (70/-); 110, 20. A 16-gauge IV catheter was inserted and an LR infusion was started. The triage nurse obtained the following history from the patient and his wife. C.W. has had idiopathic dilated cardiomyopathy (IDCM) for several years. The onset was insidious but the cardiomyopathy is now severe, as evidenced by a L ventricular ejection fraction of 13% found during a recent cardiac catheterization. He experiences frequent problems with CHF because of the IDCM. Two years ago he had a cardiac arrest that was attributed to hypokalemia. He also has a long history of hypertension and arthritis. Fifteen years ago, he had a peptic ulcer.

An endoscopy showed a 25 x 15 mm duodenal ulcer with adherent clot. The ulcer was cauterized and C.W. was admitted to the MICU for treatment of his volume deficit. You are his admitting nurse. As you are making him comfortable, Mrs. W. gives you a paper sack filled with the bottles of medications he has been taking: enalopril (Vasotec) 5 mg PO bid, warfarin (Coumadin) 5 mg PO qd, digoxin 0.125 mg PO qd, KCl 20 mEq PO bid, and tolmetin (an NSAID) 400 mg PO tid. As you connect him to the cardiac monitor, you note that he is in A fib. Doing a quick assessment, you find a pale man who is sleepy but arousable and oriented. He is still dizzy, hypotensive, and tachycardic. You hear S_3 and S_4 heart sounds and a grade II/VI systolic murmur. Peripheral pulses are all 2+ and trace pedal edema is present. Lungs are clear. Bowel sounds are present, midepigastric tenderness is noted, and the liver margin is 4 cm below the costal margin. A Swan-Ganz catheter and an arterial line are inserted.

1. What medication probably precipitated C.W.'s GI bleeding?

2. What is the most serious potential complication of C.W.'s bleeding?

3. From his history and assessment, identify five s/s (direct and/or indirect) of GI bleeding and loss of blood volume.

C.W. receives a total of 4 units of RBCs, 5 units of fresh frozen plasma (FFP), and many liters of crystalloids to keep his systolic BP above 90 mm Hg. On the second day in the MICU, his total fluid intake is 8.498 L and output 3.660 L for a positive fluid balance of 4.838 L. His hemodynamic parameters after fluid resuscitation are PCWP 30 mm Hg, CO 4.5 L/min.

4. Why will you want to monitor his fluid status very carefully?

5. List six things you will monitor to assess C.W.'s fluid balance.

6. Explain the purpose of the FFP for C.W.

As soon as you get a chance, you look at C.W.'s admission lab results: K 6.2 mmol/L, BUN 90 mg/dL, creatinine 2.1 mg/dL, Hgb 8.4 g/dL, Hct 25%, WBC 16 thou/cmm, and PT 23.4/INR = 4.2. Other results are within the normal range.

7. Are you worried by the elevated K? Why, or why not? Explain your answer.

8. In view of the elevated K, what diagnostic test should be performed and why?

9. Why do you think BUN and creatinine are elevated?

10. What do the low Hb and Hct levels indicate about the rapidity of C.W.'s blood loss?

11. What is the explanation for the prolonged PT/INR?

12. What should be your response to the prolonged PT/INR?

13. What safety precautions should be considered in light of his prolonged PT/INR?

14. How do you account for the elevated WBC count?

Mrs. W. has been with her husband since he arrived at the ED and is very worried about his condition and his care.

15. List four things you might do to make her more comfortable while her husband is in the MICU.

Case Study 18

Name ______________________ Class/Group ______ Date ______

Group Members ______________________

INSTRUCTIONS: All questions apply to this case study. Your responses should be brief and to the point. Adequate space has been provided for answers. When asked to provide several answers, they should be listed in order of priority or significance. Do not assume information that is not provided. Please print or write clearly. If your response is not legible, it will be marked as ? and you will need to rewrite it.

Scenario

K.K., a 40-year-old administrative secretary, lost consciousness and slumped to the floor while eating dinner with her husband. He initiated CPR. Paramedics arrived within 4 to 5 minutes and found her in V fib. After successful defibrillation, she was transported to the hospital. In the MICU her nurse obtained K.K.'s health history from her husband. She has a long history of rheumatic heart disease (RHD) with mitral valve prolapse (MVP) and severe L ventricular dysfunction. She has had A fib/atrial flutter for 6 years. She also has had ventricular dysrhythmias for several years being treated with various antidysrhythmic drugs and furosemide; however, she was not taking her medications at the time of the arrest because she didn't like the side effects. Her doctor feels she has been noncompliant with her medications and that she is denying her need for mitral valve replacement. For the past 2 months she has had CHF with greatly decreased activity tolerance. Medications she was taking at the time of the arrest were furosemide 80 mg PO qd, KCl 20 mEq PO bid, digoxin 0.125 mg PO qd, lisinopril 5 mg PO qd, and warfarin (Coumadin) 2.5 mg PO qd. On the day of her arrest, she had diarrhea.

1. From K.K.'s history, what factors probably contributed to her cardiac arrest?

On admission to the MICU, K.K. is hypotensive and unresponsive to voice commands. She is intubated and placed on mechanical ventilation. A central line is inserted, and dopamine and lidocaine drips are started. For the first day in the MICU, she remains unresponsive to commands, her pupillary reaction is sluggish, eyes deviate slowly to the right, upper extremities have increased tone, and lower extremities are flaccid. Painful stimuli elicit withdrawal and decorticate posturing. Her 12-lead ECG shows A fib at a rate of 136/min; ST segment depression in leads II, III, AVF, and V_1–V_6; and T wave inversion in leads V_3–V_5.

2. What is the probable cause for her neurologic deficits?

3. Explain how rapid A fib can cause a decrease in CO and contribute to CHF.

4. What is the significance of the ST segment depression and T wave inversion in her 12-lead ECG?

5. List eight lab results that the MICU nurse should check as soon as possible.

After 4 days in the MICU, K.K.'s condition is stabilized and she is transferred to your telemetry floor. When you first assess her, you find jugular vein distention at 10 cm and hear a grade II/VI systolic murmur and an S_3 sound. A thrill is felt over the precordium, and the S_1 and S_2 can be seen on the chest. She no longer has sensory or motor deficits, and her long-term memory is good. However, she is confused, oriented only to name, and has poor short-term memory. Her lidocaine level in the MICU the day before the transfer (the day the lidocaine was discontinued) was 16.8 mg/L; digoxin level was normal. A cardiac catheterization and ECHO cardiogram showed that K.K. has irreversible heart valve, L ventricle, and L atrium damage and is no longer a candidate for mitral valve replacement. She states she is very fearful about her memory loss and the inoperable heart damage. (K.K. may also be considered as a candidate for a transplant.)

6. List three factors that might be contributing to K.K.'s confusion and disorientation.

7. List four nursing interventions you might implement to relieve K.K.'s fear.

After 2 weeks in the hospital, K.K. is scheduled for placement of an internal cardioverter defibrillator (ICD or AICD) to prevent future cardiac arrest from ventricular fibrillation. You will do her preoperative teaching about ICDs.

8. What is an ICD and how does it work?

9. List four discharge instructions r/t the ICD that you will give K.K.

Case Study 19

Name ____________________________ Class/Group ______ Date ______

Group Members ____

INSTRUCTIONS: All questions apply to this case study. Your responses should be brief and to the point. Adequate space has been provided for answers. When asked to provide several answers, they should be listed in order of priority or significance. Do not assume information that is not provided. Please print or write clearly. If your response is not legible, it will be marked as ? and you will need to rewrite it.

Scenario

During a routine checkup, D.A.'s doctor heard 2 new heart murmurs: a grade II/VI diastolic flow murmur heard at the R sternal border and a prominent grade IV/VI systolic ejection murmur heard over the entire precordium but best at the L sternal border. The murmurs are asymptomatic. D.A. is a slender, active 50-year-old engineer, married with 2 teenage children. He has polycystic kidney disease with renal failure and has been on dialysis for 5 years. His mother also had polycystic kidney disease. Besides frequent UTIs, he has no other significant medical problems, no history of cardiac disease, and no cardiac risk factors. A transthoracic/transesophageal ECHO showed a "high pressure jet from the R atrium or R ventricle." Cardiac catheterization showed an "aortic to R ventricle connection through a R coronary sinus of Valsalva leak." The catheterization also showed normal coronary arteries, normal L ventricular function, and no aortic regurgitation.

D.A. was admitted to the hospital for surgical repair of a ruptured sinus of Valsalva aneurysm. During the surgery a 4-mm hole from the R coronary sinus to the R atrium was discovered and repaired with a patch. There were no complications. You are caring for D.A. in the SICU after the surgery. On the first postop day his VS are 90/54, 87, 12, 37.8° C. Central venous pressure averages 10 mm Hg. He has a temporary pacemaker set at 87/min, which is functioning correctly. Lungs are clear. He has been extubated and is on O_2 at 2 L/min by nasal cannula with an SaO_2 of 99%. He has a chest tube and indwelling urinary catheter. You review his lab results, noting BUN 120 mg/dL, creatinine 8.5 mg/dL, and K 6.2 mmol/L. His preop Hct was 32%; today it is 22.1%, and Hgb is 9.0 g/dL. Other lab values are within normal ranges.

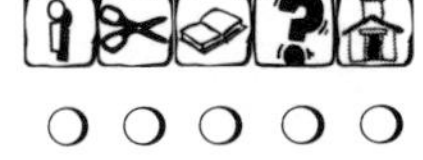

1. Which of the above physiologic data should cause you concern and prompt careful monitoring on your part?

2. When you perform your physical assessment, you should pay special attention to s/s r/t D.A.'s problems. List at least five priority assessment areas, and explain why they are important.

3. Mrs. A. is present at the bedside, supportive and anxious. Considering her apprehension, what can you do to make her more comfortable?

On the third postop day, D.A. has an infectious disease consult. The consulting physician writes in the chart, "The *Enterobacter* infection of the sinus of Valsalva is the likely cause of the aneurysm. The heart was probably seeded from a renal source. If the patch continues to harbor organisms, the patient may have future problems." D.A. was started on IV antibiotics (gentamicin and cefotaxime—ATB depends on C&S).

4. List at least three problems D.A. might have as a result of the heavy-duty antibiotic therapy. What will you monitor for each? Consider his renal failure and common side effects of the medications.

5. Mrs. A. confides in you, "You know, my 15-year-old son refuses to talk about his dad's illness. He won't even come to see him in the hospital. The guidance counselor called from school yesterday and said he's been acting out in school. I'm exhausted trying to work family life from both ends." How are you going to respond?

6. In preparation for discharge, a peripherally inserted central catheter (PICC) is placed. What is a PICC, and what are the advantages and disadvantages of this type of catheter?

D.A. is being discharged to home, where a home care nurse will continue to monitor the IV site and teach the wife how to administer the IV antibiotics.

7. Identify at least three important nursing care problems that would apply to IV antibiotic administration in the home.

Case Study 20

Name ______________________ Class/Group ______ Date ______

Group Members ______________________________________

INSTRUCTIONS: All questions apply to this case study. Your responses should be brief and to the point. Adequate space has been provided for answers. When asked to provide several answers, they should be listed in order of priority or significance. Do not assume information that is not provided. Please print or write clearly. If your response is not legible, it will be marked as ? and you will need to rewrite it.

Scenario

You are in the middle of your shift in the CCU of a large urban medical center. Your new admission, C.B., a 47-year-old woman, has just been flown in to your institution from a small rural community over 100 miles away. She is unstable after an acute MI. C.B.'s VS are 100/60, 86, 14. After you make C.B. comfortable, you receive this report from the flight nurse: "C.B. is a full-time homemaker with 4 children. She has had episodes of 'chest tightness' for several years, but this is her first documented MI. She has elevated cholesterol and triglyceride levels and has smoked 1 pack of cigarettes per day for 30 years. She had a TAH 10 years ago after the birth of her last child. Besides this, she doesn't report any other medical problems. Yesterday at 2000 she began having substernal chest pain that radiated to her neck bilaterally and down both arms. She rated the pain as 9 on a scale of 1 to 10. She lay down with a heating pad, but the pain didn't go away. Her husband then took her to the local ED, where a 12-lead ECG showed hyperacute ST elevation. They were about to give her some tPA when she went into V fib and arrested. She was successfully defibrillated with 2 shocks. Then she was given the tPA and put on lidocaine, heparin, and nitroglycerin drips. They also gave her some metoprolol. This morning when her systolic pressure dropped into the 80s, she was put on a dopamine drip and flown here for a possible percutaneous transluminal coronary angioplasty (PTCA). Right now the lidocaine is going at 2 mg/min, the heparin at 1200 µ/h, and the dopamine at 5 µ/kg/min. The nitroglycerin is off."

The flight nurse hands you a copy of yesterday's 12-lead ECG that shows normal sinus rhythm with ST elevation in leads II, III, AVF, and V_5–V_6. She also gives you a copy of yesterday's lab work: Na 145 mmol/L, K 3.6 mmol/L, HCO_3 19 mmol/L, BUN 9 mg/dL, creatinine 0.8 mg/dL, WBC 14.5 thou/cmm, Hct 44.3%, and Hgb 14.5 g/dL.

1. Given the diagnosis of acute MI, what other lab results are you going to look at?

2. You find the following lab results in the patient's chart. For each, interpret the result, and evaluate the meaning for C.B.

   a. CKs drawn upon admission to the ED and at 4-hour intervals were 95 U/L, 1931 U/L, and 4175 U/L. CK-MB isoenzymes were 5%, 79%, and 216%.

   b. Cholesterol: 180 mg/dL.

   c. SaO_2 on O_2 at 6 L/min by nasal cannula: >90%.

   d. PT was 11.9 secs/INR = 1.02, and PTT was 26.9 secs (before heparin infusion).

   e. Mg level was 2.2 mg/dL.

3. The 12-lead ECG can tell you the location of the infarction. Look at the leads that show ST elevation (see flight nurse's report). What areas of C.B.'s heart have been damaged?

4. What is tPA? Why is it given, and when is it given to a patient having an MI? How is it administered?

5. An hour after her admission, you are preparing C.B. for her PTCA. Evaluate her readiness for teaching and her learning needs. What would you tell her?

The following day you care for C.B. again. During her PTCA procedure yesterday, a circumflex coronary lesion was found and the artery was successfully dilated. She is still on the lidocaine and heparin drips. The dopamine has been discontinued. VS are stable. PCWP is 20 mm Hg, and CO is 7.3 L/min. You check her lab results for lidocaine and PTT levels.

6. The lidocaine level is 2.5 μg/ml, and the PTT is 61 seconds. Analyze the results and state any actions you would take.

As you work with C.B., you notice that she is extremely anxious. You had observed some anxiety yesterday, which you had attributed to the strange CCU environment, pain, and anticipation of the PTCA procedure. You know that the PTCA was successful and that she is physically stable. You wonder what is wrong. She tells you that her MI occurred right in the middle of a move with her family from her rural community to an even smaller and unfamiliar town some 500 miles away in a neighboring state. She is dreading the move. Her husband "becomes angry easily and starts lashing out" toward her and the children. She is afraid to move to a community where she will have no friends and family to support her.

7. How can you help your patient? Evaluate the situation and describe possible interventions.

8. C.B.'s husband comes to visit. He is a handsome, well-dressed man who appears to be loving and attentive toward C.B. He brought a bouquet of roses for her and a box of chocolates for the nurses, "Because I appreciate how good you girls have been to my wife." One of your younger colleagues comments to you, "Why, what a nice guy! What is her problem? Every woman would love to be married to a man like that!" How are you going to respond?

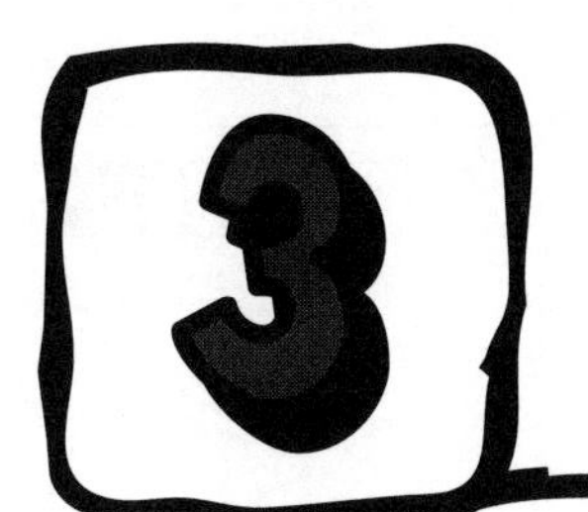

Pulmonary Disorders

Case Study 1

Name ______________________ Class/Group ______ Date ______

Group Members ____

INSTRUCTIONS: All questions apply to this case study. Your responses should be brief and to the point. Adequate space has been provided for answers. When asked to provide several answers, they should be listed in order of priority or significance. Do not assume information that is not provided. Please print or write clearly. If your response is not legible, it will be marked as ? and you will need to rewrite it.

Scenario

A.K. is a 38-year-old woman who runs 3 miles every morning. She comes to the Family Nurse Practitioner Clinic c/o a burning feeling in her throat and upper airway that begins shortly after she starts running. A.K. states that she gets increasingly more winded and sometimes has to stop running to catch her breath.

1. As the intake nurse working in the clinic, what routine information would you want to obtain from A.K.?

2. What two body systems do you suspect might be involved in A.K.'s problem?

3. What would you do to differentiate between problems in the two body systems?

You assess A.K. and note the following: S_1S_2 with no murmurs, clicks, or rubs; on inspiration her heart rate speeds up and you think you hear a split S_2; on expiration her heart rate slows down and you don't hear the split.

4. Discuss the significance of these findings. ❍ ❍ ❍ ❍ ❍

Her lungs are clear throughout and percuss resonance. You measure height and weight to calculate her estimated peak expiratory flow rate (PEFR). You then measure A.K.'s actual PEFR using a peak flow meter (PFM).

5. Explain the purpose of the PEFR measurement. ❍ ❍ ❍ ❍ ❍

6. You record A.K.'s PEFR measurement and note that it is within 5% of estimated normal PEFR. Discuss the significance of her pulmonary evaluation and these findings. ❍ ❍ ❍ ❍ ❍

The FNP confirms your examination findings and, after reviewing A.K.'s PEFR measurements, discusses the possibility of exercise-induced asthma (EIA) with A.K. She directs A.K. to record her PEFR then go for her usual morning run. If she experiences the burning feeling in her throat and upper airway and/or becomes SOB, she should stop running and immediately measure and record her PEFR. Repeat measurements should be taken at 5-minute intervals for 20 to 30 minutes. Ask A.K. to bring her PEFR record with her next time.

7. What is the FNP hoping to learn from the presymptom-to-postsymptom PEFR measurement?

A.K. returns in 1 week for a follow-up visit. She hands you a list of PEFR measurements. You calculate that A.K.'s postrun measurements range from 75% to 85% of her prerun values and her PEFR returned to normal within 25 minutes of stopping activity.

8. What does this pattern of change indicate?

The FNP gives A.K. an albuterol (Ventolin) metered-dose inhaler (MDI) with a spacer and instructs her to take 2 puffs 15 minutes before she exercises. The FNP is called to see another patient and asks you to complete the discharge teaching with A.K.

9. What information about the drug and its administration should you discuss with her?

10. A.K. says she doesn't like to be dependent on medication. How would you respond to this statement?

11. A.K. asks whether it is possible for her to develop full-blown asthma. How would you respond?

A.K. was motivated to take her MDI so that she could maintain her exercise regimen. At a follow-up visit, she tells you she saw, "Lots of folks using an MDI at last Saturday's race."

Notes: (1) Be sure you ask A.K. about frequency of MDI use each time she visits. (2) Persistent and progressive asthma should be an indication for allergy evaluation.

Case Study 2

Name ____________________ Class/Group ______ Date ______

Group Members ______________________________

INSTRUCTIONS: All questions apply to this case study. Your responses should be brief and to the point. Adequate space has been provided for answers. When asked to provide several answers, they should be listed in order of priority or significance. Do not assume information that is not provided. Please print or write clearly. If your response is not legible, it will be marked as ? and you will need to rewrite it.

M.N., age 40, is admitted with acute cholecystitis, elevated WBC, and a fever of 102° F. She has undergone an open cholecystectomy and has been transferred to your floor. It is the second day postop. She has an NGT to continuous low wall suction, one peripheral IV, and a large abdominal dressing. Her orders are as follows: progress diet to decreased fat diet as tolerated; $D_5\frac{1}{2}$NS with 40 mEq KCl at 125 ml an hour; turn, cough, and deep breathe q2h; incentive spirometer (IS) q2h while awake; dangle in AM, ambulate in PM; morphine sulfate 10 mg IM q4h for pain; ampicillin (Omnipen) 2 g IVPB q6h; chest x-ray (CXR) in AM.

1. Are these orders appropriate for M.N.? State your rationale.

2. What GI complication may result from one of the medications listed in M.N.'s orders?

   Constipation – Morphine

3. Identify the two most common respiratory-related complications for patients with abdominal or thoracic surgery.

   – SOB
   ↑RR (fever)

4. What information and assessments would help you differentiate between the two complications in question 3?

5. What procedure is necessary to differentiate between atelectasis and pneumonia?

6. You are assigned to take care of M.N. Her VS are 148/82, 118, 24, 101° F. Her SaO_2 is 88%. Based on these numbers, what do you think is going on with M.N. and why?

Bleeding

7. You know M.N. is at risk for postop atelectasis. What is atelectasis?

After morning report, you do an assessment and auscultate decreased breath sounds and crackles in the R base posteriorally. Her RML and RLL percuss slightly dull. She splints her R side when attempting to take a deep breath. You suspect that she is developing atelectasis.

8. What most likely accounts for M.N.'s inspiratory-related behavior?

9. What effect will M.N.'s splinting have on potential atelectasis?

10. Identify and clarify five actions you would take next.

11. What four interventions might be used to prevent pulmonary complications?

O_2

12. Identify three outcomes that you expect for M.N. as a result of your nursing interventions and her increased activity?

13. M.N.'s sister questions you, saying, “I don't understand. She came in here with a bad gallbladder. What has happened to her lungs?” How would you respond?

14. Radiology calls up with a report from the radiologist on the AM CXR. M.N. has atelectasis. Will that change anything that you have already planned for M.N.? Explain what you would do differently if M.N. had pneumonia.

Case Study 4

Name ______________________ Class/Group ______ Date ______

Group Members ____

INSTRUCTIONS: All questions apply to this case study. Your responses should be brief and to the point. Adequate space has been provided for answers. When asked to provide several answers, they should be listed in order of priority or significance. Do not assume information that is not provided. Please print or write clearly. If your response is not legible, it will be marked as ? and you will need to rewrite it.

Scenario

P.R., a 31-year-old woman, contracted an upper respiratory tract infection, developed a high fever, and began to experience progressive ascending paralysis. She was admitted to the local hospital, diagnosed with Guillain-Barré syndrome. She was intubated and mechanically ventilated. Her VS are 112/68, 134, 12, 101° F. The placement of her PEG tube was confirmed by abdominal x-ray. Her total parenteral nutrition (TPN) was discontinued yesterday, and she was started on enteral nutrition (EN). The consulting dietitian calculated P.R.'s caloric need at 2800 calories/24 hours. P.R. is 5'4" and weighs 123 lb. (Note: Registered dietitians prefer the "t" spelling rather than "dietician.")

1. What is ascending paralysis?

2. Identify and discuss at least two factors that would influence the physician's decision to place P.R. on EN.

3. Is 2800 kcal/24 hr a normal caloric requirement for a woman 5'4", 123 lb? Compare her provided EN caloric needs with the "ideal" values for a woman of her height and weight. Is it higher or lower? Explain the reason for her current needs.

4. Absolute medical contraindications to enteral feeding are few, and it is preferable to demonstrate failure of EN than to assume that the GI tract is nonfunctional and initiate TPN. Give three examples of medical diagnoses for which EN would be contraindicated.

5. Pulmonary aspiration is a risk with enteral feedings, although the risk is substantially reduced with duodenal placement. Identify four measures that can be taken to minimize the risk for aspiration.

6. Identify five strategies for preventing bacterial contamination of the feeding formula and tubing.

7. Identify two indicators that an EN infusion rate is too rapid.

8. The nurse needs to monitor P.R.'s GI response to EN and steroid therapy. Identify two observations that need to be recorded, and explain the significance of each.

9. It is a common belief that diarrhea (defined as >3 liquid stools per day) is a natural consequence of EN administration. Discuss whether this is a true statement.

10. Identify three factors that could cause diarrhea.

As P.R.'s nurse, you are concerned about meeting her needs for fluids, oral hygiene, skin integrity, and activity.

11. Discuss five indicators that would help you assess fluid status.

12. The goal r/t P.R.'s mouth care is to preserve the oral mucosa and dentition. Identify three strategies for providing oral hygiene with an oral endotracheal tube (ETT) in place.

13. What is the rationale for not taking an oral temperature near an ETT?

14. You assess P.R.'s skin every 4 hours. Identify three treatment goals in relation to skin/positioning.

15. What four strategies will facilitate the expected outcome of maintaining skin integrity?

16. You approach P.R. to begin ROM exercises. You ask her whether she is experiencing muscle pain at this time and she nods "yes." You tell P.R. that you will wait until she is pain-free to perform the exercises. Why?

It takes nearly a year for P.R. to make a full recovery.

Case Study 5

Name ____________________ Class/Group ______ Date ______

Group Members ____________________________________

INSTRUCTIONS: All questions apply to this case study. Your responses should be brief and to the point. Adequate space has been provided for answers. When asked to provide several answers, they should be listed in order of priority or significance. Do not assume information that is not provided. Please print or write clearly. If your response is not legible, it will be marked as ? and you will need to rewrite it.

Scenario

M.N., a 22-year-old man, who lives in a small mountain town in Colorado, is highly allergic to dust and pollen; anxiety appears to play a role in exacerbating his asthma attacks. M.N.'s wife drove him to the clinic when his wheezing was unresponsive to beclomethasone (Vanceril) and ipratropium bromide (Atrovent) inhalers. Upon arrival, his VS are 152/84, 124, 42, 100.4° F. M.N. is started on 4 L O_2/nc, an IV of D_5W at KVO. His ABGs are pH 7.31, $PaCO_2$ 48 mmHg, HCO_3 26 mmol/L, PaO_2 55 mmHg, SaO_2 88%.

1. Explain the pathophysiology of asthma.

2. Identify pathophysiologic responses during an asthma attack.

3. Are M.N.'s VS acceptable? State your rationale.

4. Comment on M.N.'s SaO_2.

5. Identify the drug classifications and actions of Vanceril and Atrovent.

6. Are Vanceril and/or Atrovent appropriate for use during an asthma attack? Explain.

7. The physician orders albuterol 3 mg nebulization treatment STAT. What is the rationale for this order?

8. What is the rationale for immediately starting M.N. on oxygen?

9. List five short-term interventions that may help relieve M.N.'s symptoms.

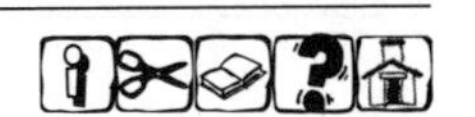

After several hours of IV and PO rehydration and a second albuterol treatment, M.N.'s wheezing and chest tightness resolve, and he is able to expectorate his secretions. The doctor discusses M.N.'s asthma management with him, and he tells him that his inhalers meet his needs on a day-to-day basis but fail him when he has an asthma attack. The doctor discharges M.N. with a prescription for Proventil MDI and a "spacer" and recommends that he call the pulmonary clinic for follow-up with a pulmonary specialist.

10. What issues would you address in discharge teaching with M.N.? ❍ ❍ ❍ ❍ ❍

You ask M.N. to demonstrate the use of his MDI. He vigorously shakes the canister, holds the aerosolizer at an angle (pointing toward his cheek) in front of his mouth, and squeezes the canister as he takes a quick, deep breath.

11. What common mistakes has M.N. made when using the inhaler? ❍ ❍ ❍ ❍ ❍

12. What would you teach M.N. about the use of his MDI? ❍ ❍ ❍ ❍ ❍

Give him written instructions about follow-up with the pulmonary specialist, and instruct him, in writing, to ask the pulmonary doctor about a "peak flow meter" (PFM).

13. What is the function of a peak flow meter (PFM), and how is it used?

14. M.N.'s wife asks about the possibility of M.N. having another attack. How would you respond?

People with a history of asthma often have special problems with postoperative care. Anesthesia can exacerbate their asthma.

15. If you have a postoperative patient with a history of asthma, what early s/s would indicate respiratory distress? (List at least six.)

Tip: To hear lung sounds better, first have the patient turn her or his head to the side (i.e., not facing you) and cough prior to auscultating.

Case Study 6

Name ______________________ Class/Group ______ Date ______

Group Members ______________________________________

INSTRUCTIONS: All questions apply to this case study. Your responses should be brief and to the point. Adequate space has been provided for answers. When asked to provide several answers, they should be listed in order of priority or significance. Do not assume information that is not provided. Please print or write clearly. If your response is not legible, it will be marked as ? and you will need to rewrite it.

Scenario

J.D., a 38-year-old man, is admitted to your medical floor with a diagnosis of pleural effusion. He c/o SOB, pain in his chest, and weakness. His VS are 142/82, 118, 38 (labored and shallow), 102° F. His CXR shows a large pleural effusion and pulmonary infiltrates in the right lower lobe (RLL) consistent with pneumonitis. (Note: When the cause of the lung infection is unknown, the condition should be referred to as *pneumonitis*.)

1. Given his diagnosis, are J.D.'s admission VS expected? Explain.

HR = 118
RR = 38
T = 102

Clinical manifestation of pleural effusion are dyspnea, fever,

2. How does his increased metabolic rate r/t his nutritional needs? Clarify.

fast breathing — fluid
RR = 38 → looses CO_2 → becoming Respiratory alkalosis

3. What is pleural effusion?

✓

4. List three common causes of pleural effusion.

✓

5. Review the pathophysiology and consequences of pleural effusion and pulmonary infiltrates. ❍ ❍ ❍ ❍ ❍

6. What is the difference between exudate and transudate? ❍ ❍ ❍ ❍ ❍

blood vessel leak holes are big The same as blood

only watery fluid

7. How does the underlying pathophysiology give rise to the presenting s/s? ❍ ❍ ❍ ❍ ❍

There is a collection of fluid in the pleural space This attracts the growth of bacteria → fever

The physician performs a thoracentesis and drains 1500 ml fluid. A specimen for C&S is sent to the laboratory, and the patient is started on cefuroxime 1 g IVPB q8h. Cephalosporins – 2nd generation

8. What is a thoracentesis? ❍ ❍ ❍ ❍ ❍

A procedure done to remove fluid from the pleural space.

9. What maneuvers would promote the clearance of pulmonary secretions? ❍ ❍ ❍ ❍ ❍

Encourage pt to cough & deep breathing Change client's position frequently

10. You enter the room to reposition J.D. If he is on his back, what side would you turn him to and why?

Semi-fowler's position – to facilitate breathing

11. The pleural fluid C&S results indicate a large amount of *Klebsiella* growth that is sensitive to cefuroxime. What action should you take next?

12. Because fluid continues to collect in the pleural space, the physician decides to insert a pleural chest tube under nonemergent conditions. What is your responsibility as J.D.'s nurse?

- drainage >100 ml – notify the physician
- monitor the volume, rate & nature of drainage
- Bloody drainage is potential for clot formation in the tubing
- If clot forms, gently milk the tube to move the clot into the collection chamber

13. Evaluate each of the following statements about chest tube drainage systems. Circle "T" for true or "F" for false. Discuss why the false statements are incorrect.

a. T F It is the height of the column of water in the suction control mechanism, not the setting of the suction source, that actually limits the amount of suction transmitted to the pleural cavity.

b. T F A suction pressure of +20 cm H_2O is commonly recommended for adults.

c. T F Bubbling in the water seal chamber means that air is leaking from the lungs, the tubing, or the insertion site. F
Gentle bubbling indicates that there is suction

d. T F The rise and fall of the water level with the patient's respirations reflects normal pressure changes in the pleural cavity with respirations. T
inhale – water fall exhale – water rises

e. T F The chamber is a closed system; therefore water cannot evaporate.

f. T F To declot the drainage tubing, put lotion on your hands, compress the tubing, and strip long segments of the tubing before releasing. F
do not milk chest tube routinely because this ↑ pleural pressures

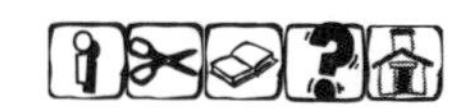

g. T F You lower the bed on top of the drainage system and break it. Because you noted an air leak from the lung during your initial assessment, you may clamp the chest tube for the short time it takes to reestablish the drainage system.

h. T F The chest tube becomes disconnected from the drainage system. Because you noted an air leak from the lung during your initial assessment, you can submerge the chest tube 1 to 2 inches below the surface of a 250 ml bottle of sterile saline or water.

i. T F The collection chamber is full so you need to connect a new drainage system to the chest tube. It is appropriate to momentarily clamp the chest tube while you disconnect the old system and reconnect the new.

j. T F The drainage system falls over, spilling the chest drainage into the other drainage columns. The total amount of drainage can be obtained by adding the amount of drainage in each of the columns.

14. Visiting hours have begun. An attractive young woman approaches you at the desk and states she is J.D.'s wife. She asks what room he is in. You know that another woman, his real wife, is already in the room with him now. How are you going to handle this? ❍ ❍ ❍ ❍ ❍

J.D. does some fast talking and manages to avoid discovery. He receives aggressive antibiotic and pulmonary therapy and is discharged 3 days later with follow-up home care.

Case Study 7

Name ______________________ Class/Group ______ Date ______

Group Members ____

INSTRUCTIONS: All questions apply to this case study. Your responses should be brief and to the point. Adequate space has been provided for answers. When asked to provide several answers, they should be listed in order of priority or significance. Do not assume information that is not provided. Please print or write clearly. If your response is not legible, it will be marked as ? and you will need to rewrite it.

❍ ❍ ❍ / ❍ ❍

Scenario

A.W., a 52-year-old woman disabled from severe emphysema, was walking at a mall when she suddenly grabbed her right side and gasped, "Oh, something just popped." A.W. whispered to her walking companion, "I can't get any air." Her companion yelled for someone to call 911 and helped her to the nearest bench. By the time the rescue unit arrived, A.W. was stuporous and in severe respiratory distress. She was intubated, an IV of LR at KVO was started, and she was transported to the nearest ED.

On arrival to the ED, the physician auscultates muffled heart tones, no breath sounds on the R, and faint sounds on the L. A.W. is stuporous, tachycardic, and cyanotic. The paramedics inform the physician that it was difficult to ventilate A.W. A STAT portable CXR and ABGs are obtained. A.W. has an 80% pneumothorax on the R, and her ABGs on 100% oxygen are pH 7.25, $PaCO_2$ 92 mmHg, PaO_2 32 mmHg, HCO_3 27 mmol/L, BE +5 mmol/L, SaO_2 53%.

1. Given the diagnosis of pneumothorax, explain why the paramedic had difficulty ventilating A.W. ❍ ❍ ❍ ❍ ❍

2. Interpret A.W.'s ABGs. ❍ ❍ ❍ ❍ ❍

3. What is the reason for A.W.'s ABG results? ❍ ❍ ❍ ❍ ❍

4. The physician needs to insert a chest tube. What are your responsibilities as the nurse?

5. As the nurse, it is your responsibility to ensure pain control. In A.W.'s case, would you administer pain medication before the chest tube insertion?

6. The ED physician inserts a size 32 chest tube in the second intercostal space, midclavicular line. Many chest tubes are inserted in the sixth intercostal space, midaxillary line. What factor determines where a chest tube is placed?

7. Given the information above, would you expect to observe an air leak when A.W.'s chest drainage system is in place and functioning?

8. Would you expect A.W.'s lung to reexpand immediately after the chest tube insertion and initiation of underwater suction? Explain.

9. The clerk tells you A.W.'s husband has just arrived; A.W. will be admitted to the hospital. How would you address this issue with her husband?

10. You approach A.W.'s bedside and ask about what looks like two healed chest tube sites on her L chest. A.W.'s husband informs you that this is the third time she has had a collapsed lung. He asks whether this trend will continue. How would you respond?

11. A.W. recovers and is discharged home 4 days later with a chest tube and Heimlich valve. The physician connects a one-way (Heimlich) valve between the distal end of the chest tube and a drainage pouch. Discuss the purpose of this device.

A.W. develops several more spontaneous pneumothoraces on the R and eventually has bleomycin instilled over the L lung to induce scarring. She says, "It felt like someone poured kerosene in and threw a lit match in after it. It was the most painful thing I ever went through." Research the scarring procedure so that you know what it does and why it is necessary.

Note: Sclerosing a lung doesn't have to feel like it is burning; it should be managed with adequate pain medication.

Case Study 8

Name ______________________ Class/Group ______ Date ______

Group Members ______________________________________

INSTRUCTIONS: All questions apply to this case study. Your responses should be brief and to the point. Adequate space has been provided for answers. When asked to provide several answers, they should be listed in order of priority or significance. Do not assume information that is not provided. Please print or write clearly. If your response is not legible, it will be marked as ? and you will need to rewrite it.

Scenario

C.K. is a very healthy, active 71-year-old who called his physician's office one day with c/o chills and cough. After taking a quick history, the nurse practitioner instructs C.K. to go to the hospital for admission. He is given a diagnosis of R/O pneumonia. The intern is busy and asks you to complete your routine admission assessment and call her with your findings. C.K. is not taking any medication and denies food or drug allergies.

1. Identify the five most important things to include in your assessment.

Your assessment findings are as follows: C.K.'s VS are 154/82, 105, 32, 103° F. You auscultate crackles in the LLL anteriorly and posteriorly. His nailbeds are dusky on fingers and toes. He has cough-productive rust-colored sputum and c/o pain in his left chest when he coughs. C.K. seems to be well-nourished and adequately hydrated. He comments that he's been "healthy as a horse" except he "got hives" when he took "one of them antibiotic pills" a few years ago.

2. Which of these assessment findings concern you? State your rationale.

The intern writes the following orders: regular diet; VS with temp q2h; maintenance IV of D_5½NS at 125 ml/h; cefuroxime (Zinacef) 1 g IVPB q8h; titrate to maintain oximeter (SaO_2) >90%; obtain sputum for culture and sensitivity (C&S) x 3; draw blood cultures x 2 sites for temp >102° F; hemogram with differential (hemogram with differential used to be known as "CBC with differential"), basic metabolic panel (basic metabolic panel, BMP, used to be referred to as the "Chem 7"), and urinalysis with C&S as indicated; CXR on admission and in the AM.

3. Review the orders and determine what you would do first.

4. Is cefuroxime appropriate for this patient? State your rationale and the significance in terms of what you should do.

5. Is the intravenous fluid of D_5½NS appropriate for C.K.? State your rationale.

6. What is the rationale for ordering oxygen to maintain SaO_2 >90%?

7. What is a culture and sensitivity test, and why is it important?

8. Why would blood cultures be drawn if the patient spikes a fever? ❍ ❍ ❍ ❍ ❍

9. Why are blood cultures drawn from two different sites? ❍ ❍ ❍ ❍ ❍

10. What general information can be obtained from a CXR? ❍ ❍ ❍ ❍ ❍

11. C.K. recovers from his pneumonia and is preparing for discharge. You know that C.K. is at increased risk for contracting community-acquired pulmonary infections. Discuss 4 strategies for prevention. ❍ ❍ ❍ ❍ ❍

12. C.K. confides in you, "You know, my wife died a year ago, and I live alone now. I've been thinking . . . this pneumonia stuff has been a little scary." How will you respond?

Note: Pneumonia, etiology unknown, is properly called "pneumonitis." When "pneumonitis" is used, it should be defined according to cause, such as viral pneumonia or *Klebsiella pneumonia*.

Case Study 9

Name ______________________ Class/Group ______ Date ______

Group Members ____

INSTRUCTIONS: All questions apply to this case study. Your responses should be brief and to the point. Adequate space has been provided for answers. When asked to provide several answers, they should be listed in order of priority or significance. Do not assume information that is not provided. Please print or write clearly. If your response is not legible, it will be marked as ? and you will need to rewrite it.

❍ ❍ ❍ / ❍ ❍

Scenario

S.M., a 67-year-old woman with severe emphysema, lives with her daughter. Six months ago, S.M. was admitted to the hospital for respiratory failure with severe hypercapnia. She received aggressive treatment with bronchodilators, mucolytics, and steroids. To improve her oxygenation, she underwent a minor surgical procedure for placement of a transtracheal (TT) catheter. She was discharged on bronchodilator and steroid therapy and continued to do well until last evening when she became profoundly SOB and had to sit in a chair all night. This morning, the admitting nurse interviews S.M. to determine why she came to the pulmonary clinic.

1. What is hypercapnia? ❍ ❍ ❍ ❍ ❍

2. S.M. has a TT O_2 catheter at 4 L/min. Describe the catheter and identify its function. ❍ ❍ ❍ ❍ ❍

3. Identify five complications associated with TT O_2 therapy. ❍ ❍ ❍ ❍ ❍

4. There is a possibility that S.M.'s TT catheter is occluded. What should the nurse do before removing the catheter for cleaning?

The nurse cleans the catheter and removes several "mucus balls." She then completes a thorough assessment and notes the following: S.M. remains very anxious after the TT O_2 catheter is cleared. Her VS are 112/72, 114, 32, 37.0° C on 4 L/O_2 per TT catheter. She is dyspneic and uses accessory muscles of the neck and abdomen for respirations. There are scattered wheezes throughout the R lung fields and LUL, rhonchi over large airways, and breath sounds are absent from fourth intercostal space to the base on L side and greatly reduced on the R. Her skin is thin and friable, with multiple ecchymoses over both arms.She has a moderate amount of hard, dark, guaiac-positive stool.

5. Based on the assessment findings, identify at least five possible problems that S.M. may be experiencing.

6. Given S.M.'s history and your knowledge of pathophysiologic processes, explain the assessment findings.

The CXR reveals LLL pneumonia. S.M. is transported to the hospital and admitted to your intermediate care unit for exacerbation of COPD and pneumonia. The doctor writes the following orders: methylprednisolone (Solu-Medrol) 40 mg IV q8h; azithromycin (Zithromax) 500 mg PO qd x 10 days; cefuroxine (Zinacef) 2g IV q6h; aerosol treatments using albuterol 2.5 mg (0.5 ml) in 3 ml NS; ranitidine (Zantac) 150 mg PO bid.

7. Describe why each of the medications is prescribed for S.M. ❍ ❍ ❍ ❍ ❍

8. While you are administering the first dose of medication, S.M. states, "I'm not gonna have that tube shoved down my throat again. I won't go on that breathing machine. I have lived with my lung disease for 30 years, and I'd rather die than live on that machine." What action(s) would you take next? State your rationale. ❍ ❍ ❍ ❍ ❍

You arrange a family conference with S.M., her daughter, the physician, and yourself. After some discussion, the physician assures S.M. that medical management will focus on resolving the pneumonia and keeping her comfortable and that her wishes regarding no resuscitation efforts will be respected. The physician details the instructions in the physician orders.

9. Describe how palliative care differs from curative care. ❍ ❍ ❍ ❍ ❍

10. Formulate a list of at least six nursing problems r/t S.M.'s care. ❍ ❍ ❍ ❍ ❍

11. Before leaving, the daughter stops you in the hallway and says, "I know that the doctor only gave my mother a couple of months to live. I know she's really sick. Is there anything I can do to make her more comfortable?" How would you respond?

Note: Also, take the opportunity to ask the daughter if a family member or significant other could relieve her so that she can get adequate rest and nutrition. Explain that she has to take care of herself before she can take care of her mother. Direct other nurses to allow the daughter to be involved in her mother's care. Place a note in the Kardex and on the patient's chart.

S.M. was discharged home with a referral for hospice care. Her daughter wrote a "Thank You" note to the nurses on your floor informing you that her mother died peacefully at home 2 weeks later.

Case Study 10

Name ____________________ Class/Group ______ Date ______

Group Members ______________________________________

INSTRUCTIONS: All questions apply to this case study. Your responses should be brief and to the point. Adequate space has been provided for answers. When asked to provide several answers, they should be listed in order of priority or significance. Do not assume information that is not provided. Please print or write clearly. If your response is not legible, it will be marked as ? and you will need to rewrite it.

Scenario

C.E., a 73-year-old married man and retired railroad engineer, visits his internist complaining: "Whenever I try to do anything, I get so out of breath I can't go on. I think I'm just getting older, but my wife told me I had to come see you about it." C.E.'s pulse oximetry (SaO_2) registers 83% at rest. He is sent to the local hospital for a CXR and ABGs to be drawn after resting 20 minutes on room air. The next day, his physician calls C.E. and informs him that he has severe emphysema and must start on continuous oxygen therapy.

1. What is C.E.'s chief complaint (CC)?

2. What is emphysema?

3. What is the most common cause of emphysema? Based on this information, what questions will you ask about health behaviors?

4. List two authoritative Internet resources of professional and patient/family information on lung disease.

5. Locate and print a patient-education handout in Spanish *and* in English on emphysema from one of the Internet sites or a similar resource. Staple it to this assignment. ❍ ❍ ❍ ❍ ❍

The physician tells C.E. that his office will have a home health equipment company call him to make arrangements to deliver the equipment and educate him in its use. As an RN working for the company, you are assigned to make the initial home visit.

Note: Diagnosis of emphysema is usually made from the CXR and ABGs on room air. Insurance companies and Medicare usually pay for oxygen only if room air ABGs show a PaO_2 <55 mm Hg.

For further information, locate HCFA/Medicare on the Internet. Look under U.S. Department of Health and Human Services, Health Care Financing Administration, for the most recent directives.

Look up the Medicare code (number) and information on reimbursement for home treatment of severe emphysema.

6. How would you prepare for the first visit? ❍ ❍ ❍ ❍ ❍

7. What issues would you address with C.E. and his wife? ❍ ❍ ❍ ❍ ❍

8. The next time you visit, C.E. c/o sores behind his ears. He explains, "That long oxygen tubing seems to take on a life of its own. It twists around and gets caught under doors, chairs, everything. It darn near rips the ears off my head." What can you tell him that could help?

9. You auscultate C.E.'s breath sounds and detect the odor of Vicks VapoRub. When you question C.E. about the use of Vicks, he tells you that he started to apply it in and around his nose to prevent his nose from becoming dry and sore. How would you council C.E. and his wife (safety issues)?

C.E. elected to use liquid oxygen because it offers more freedom and portability. It is also lighter in weight.

10. Over the next 3 weeks, C.E. seemed to adjust well to his liquid oxygen system. However, one evening he walked to the kitchen for a snack and became increasingly SOB. Identify three possible causes.

As per your instructions, C.E. removed the nasal cannula, tested the flow against his check, and felt no oxygen flowing from the catheter. He lacked the force and volume required to yell for help and was too SOB to return to the living room to check his oxygen tank. He bent forward with his elbows on the counter top, and struggled to breathe. He became more frightened with each passing second, and his breathing seemed to become increasingly more difficult. A minute later, C.E.'s wife found him and reconnected his oxygen tubing. C.E. sat at the table for 20 minutes before he could walk back to the living room.

11. Why did C.E. assume the peculiar position at the counter top? ❍ ❍ ❍ ❍ ❍

12. A week later you receive a call from C.E.'s wife. She relates the incident from the previous week and tells you that C.E. "doesn't want her out of his sight." She asks you to come to the house and "talk some sense into him." What teaching strategies will you use with C.E. and his wife? ❍ ❍ ❍ ❍ ❍

13. C.E.'s wife asks you what her husband can do to help her around the house. She says, "The doctor told him to go home and take it easy. He sits in a chair all day. He won't even get up to get himself a glass of water. I've got a bad hip and this has been very hard on me." How would you address her issue? ❍ ❍ ❍ ❍ ❍

An OT instructs the couple about energy saving ways to complete their housework. They both seem satisfied with their new division of labor. In addition, the women's group at their church has volunteered to help once a week with laundry, vacuuming, and other stressful tasks.

14. C.E. states, "You seem to know what you are talking about, so let me ask you something. I wake up with a headache almost every morning. My wife says it's because I snore so loud and don't breathe right when I sleep. Do you know anything about that?" After asking several questions, you inform C.E. that it sounds like he has obstructive sleep apnea. Explain the connection between obstructive sleep apnea and morning headaches. ❍ ❍ ❍ ❍ ❍

15. C.E. seems impressed by your explanation. He asks whether there is anything that can be done for his problem. You inform him that there is a treatment called continuous positive airway pressure (CPAP). What is CPAP, and how does it work? What is the difference between CPAP and BiPAP? ❍ ❍ ❍ ❍ ❍

You comment that C.E. sounds like he has a cold. He replies, "Oh, our great-grandchildren were over to visit several days ago and they all had snotty noses. I suspect that I'll get it pretty soon. The problem is, every time I get a cold it goes straight to my lungs."

16. What information would you want to review with C.E. and his wife about the s/s of infection and when to seek treatment? ❍ ❍ ❍ ❍ ❍

17. What basic hygiene measures can C.E. and his wife take to prevent his developing an infection? (List at least four.)

18. Why is it important for people with lung disease to seek early intervention for infection?

C.E. seemed to be managing his emphysema fairly well. His wife had her hip replaced, made a speedy recovery, and was discharged to home. She suddenly died 4 weeks later from a pulmonary embolus. C.E. was panic-stricken at her loss. A psychiatric nurse practitioner was requested to work with him.

Note: It is important to keep in mind that many home-bound people with chronic illnesses are living a fragile functional independence, depending on the assistance of their partner. When something happens to the partner (death, illness, or stress-related illnesses), the remaining person is often forced into a nursing home. It is also easier to understand the pressures experienced by the assisting partner: stress-related illnesses, alcoholism, and other forms of substance abuse are not uncommon in these settings, especially where poor community support and inadequate symptom management are factors.

Case Study 11

Name ________________ Class/Group ______ Date ______

Group Members ________________________________

INSTRUCTIONS: All questions apply to this case study. Your responses should be brief and to the point. Adequate space has been provided for answers. When asked to provide several answers, they should be listed in order of priority or significance. Do not assume information that is not provided. Please print or write clearly. If your response is not legible, it will be marked as ? and you will need to rewrite it.

Scenario

The ICU nurse calls to give you the following report: "D.S. is a 56-year-old man with a PMH of chronic bronchitis. He quit smoking 12 years ago and exercises regularly. He went to see his doc with c/o increasing exertional dyspnea; a large mass was found in his R lung. Three days ago he underwent an RML and RLL lobectomy; the pathology report showed adenocarcinoma. He has no neuro deficits and his VS run 120s/70s, 110s, about 34, and he has been running a fever of 100.2° F. His heart tones are clear, he has all his pulses, and has an IV of D_5½NS at 50 ml/h in his R forearm. He has a R midaxillary chest tube to PleurEvac drain; there's no air leak, and it's draining small amounts of serosanguinous fluid. He's c/o pain at the insertion site, but the site looks good, and the dressing is dry and intact. He's on 5 L O_2. He refuses pain medication. He's a real nervous guy and hasn't slept since surgery. He'll be there in about 20 minutes."

1. What additional information would you ask the nurse to provide at this time?

D.S. is transported by wheelchair past the nurses' station to a room at the far end of the hall. You enter his room for the first time to find him sitting on the edge of the bed with his left leg in bed and his right foot on the floor. You introduce yourself and tell him that you are going to be his nurse for the rest of the shift. You note that he keeps rubbing his left hand over his right chest.

2. What issues/problems can you already identify?

3. List four things you would do for D.S. ❍ ❍ ❍ ❍ ❍

D.S. states, "I have a nephew who rolled his Jeep and busted himself up real bad. He got hooked on those drugs, and I don't want any part of them."

4. How would you respond to D.S.'s statement. ❍ ❍ ❍ ❍ ❍

5. Why is D.S. experiencing difficulty using his R arm? Given the type of surgery he underwent, is this expected? ❍ ❍ ❍ ❍ ❍

6. You administer 8 mg morphine (MSO_4) IM and tell D.S. that you will return in 30 minutes; 15 minutes later he turns on his call light. When you enter the room D.S. says, "I think I'm going to throw up." What are the next 3 things you would do?

7. D.S. stated, "I started to feel sick a couple minutes ago. It just kept getting worse until I knew I was going to throw up." Given this information, what do you think is responsible for the sudden onset of nausea?

8. Would it be appropriate to give D.S. a second dose of morphine before reporting his reaction to the physician? State your rationale.

9. D.S.'s pain and nausea are under control an hour later. You remove the chest tube dressing and note that the area around the insertion site looks slightly inflamed, the tissue immediately around the tube looks white, and there is a small amount of purulent drainage. What action would you take next?

The next day the nurse giving you report says that D.S. has been driving her crazy all day long. She tells you that he is fine but has been paranoid and very demanding. You enter D.S.'s room to see how he is doing and to tell him you are going to be his nurse again today. You note that his head bobs up and his mouth opens, like a fish taking in water, every time he inhales. He says, "I just can't [breath] seem to [breath] get enough [breath] air."

10. Identify six possible problems that D.S. could have that would account for his behavior.

11. What three actions should you take next? Give your rationale.

D.S.'s R is 46; you auscultate slight air movement over the large airways and no breath sounds distal to the third ICS. He's sitting on the side of the bed with his arms hunched up on the overbed table. His gown is in his lap, he is diaphoretic, you note intercostal retractions with inspiration, and all muscles of the upper torso are engaged in respiration.

12. What would you do next?

D.S. is successfully resuscitated and transferred to ICU. The physician returns to your floor and compliments you on your clear thinking and fast action. The nurse who gave you report comes up to you to apologize. She is relatively new and asks you to explain how you know when a patient is in the early and late stages of respiratory difficulty. She states that she wants to learn from her mistakes so that she doesn't put another patient through what D.S. experienced.

13. How would you distinguish between early and late stages of respiratory failure?

D.S. recovers. His CXR at 5 years shows no recurrence.

Case Study 12

Name ______________________ Class/Group ______ Date ______

Group Members ______________________________________

INSTRUCTIONS: All questions apply to this case study. Your responses should be brief and to the point. Adequate space has been provided for answers. When asked to provide several answers, they should be listed in order of priority or significance. Do not assume information that is not provided. Please print or write clearly. If your response is not legible, it will be marked as ? and you will need to rewrite it.

Scenario

G.S., a 36-year-old secretary, was involved in a motor vehicle accident; a car drifted left of center and struck G.S. head-on, pinning her behind the steering wheel. She was intubated immediately after extrication and flown to your trauma center. Her injuries were found to be extensive: bilateral flail chest, torn innominate artery, right hemo/pneumothorax, fractured spleen, multiple small liver lacerations, compound fractures of both legs, and probable cardiac contusion. She was taken to the OR where she received 36 units of PRCs, 20 units of platelets, 20 units cryoprecipitate, 12 units FFP, and 18 L of LR. She was admitted to the intensive care unit (ICU) postop where she developed adult respiratory distress syndrome (ARDS). She has been in ICU for 6 weeks, and her ARDS has almost resolved. She is transferred to your unit. You receive the following report: Neuro: AAO to person and place, she can move both of her arms and wiggle her toes on both feet; CV: heart tones are clear, VS are 138/90, 88, 26, 99.2° F, bilateral radial pulse 3+, foot pulses by Doppler only; Skin: incisions and lacerations have all healed; Respiratory: bilateral chest tubes to water suction with closed drainage, dressings are dry and intact; GI: duodenal feeding tube in place; GU: Foley catheter to down drain.

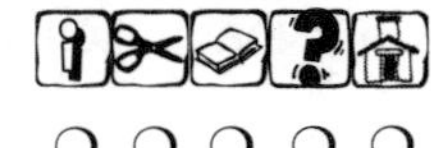
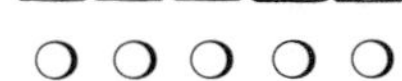

1. What additional information should you require during this report?

You complete your assessment of G.S. You note SOB, crackles throughout all lung fields posteriorally and in both lower lobes anteriorly, and rhonchi over the large airways.

2. What is the significance of crackles and rhonchi in G.S.'s case?

3. The nurse from the previous shift charted the following statement, "Crackles and rhonchi clear with vigorous coughing." Based on your knowledge of pathophysiology, determine the accuracy of this statement.

4. It is time to administer 40 mg furosemide (Lasix) IVP. What effect, if any, will Lasix have on G.S.'s breath sounds?

5. What action should you take before giving the Lasix?

The 0500 laboratory values are as follows: Na 129 mmol/L, K 3.3 mmol/L, Cl 92 mmol/L, HCO_3 26 mmol/L, BUN 37 mg/dL, creatinine 2.0 mg/dL, glucose 128 mg/dL, calcium 7.1 mg/dL, ABGs on 6 L O_2/nc: pH 7.38, $PaCO_2$ 49 mm Hg, PaO_2 82 mm Hg, HCO_3 36 mmol/L, BE +2.2, SaO_2 91%.

6. Keeping in mind that you are about to administer Lasix, which laboratory values concern you and why?

7. Given the laboratory values listed, what action would you take before administering the furosemide, and why? ❍ ❍ ❍ ❍ ❍

The physician prescribes the following: draw STAT Mg level; if below 1.4 mg/dL, give $MgSO_4$ 3 g in 100 ml D_5W over 4h; give KCl 40 mEq in 100 ml D_5W IVPB over 4h NOW; and give $CaCl_2$ g in 100 ml D_5W IVPB over 3h. The laboratory is called to draw a STAT Mg level.

8. Given that KCl and CaCl are compatible, would you mix them in the same bag of D_5W? State your rationale. ❍ ❍ ❍ ❍ ❍

9. You open G.S.'s medication drawer to draw the Lasix into a syringe. You find one 20-mg ampule. The pharmacist tells you that it will be at least an hour before he can send the drug to you. You realize it is illegal to take medication dispensed by a pharmacist for one patient and use it for another patient. What should you do? ❍ ❍ ❍ ❍ ❍

10. While you administer the Lasix and hang the IVPB medication, G.S. says, "This is so weird. A couple times this morning, I felt like my heart flipped upside down in my chest, but now I feel like there's a bird flopping around in there." What are the first two actions you should take next? Give your rationale. ❍ ❍ ❍ ❍ ❍

11. G.S.'s pulse is 66 and irregular. Her BP is 92/70, and respirations are 26. She admits to being "a little light-headed" but denies having pain or nausea. Your coworker connects G.S. to the code cart monitor for a "quick look." You are able to distinguish normal P-QRS-T complexes, but you also note approximately 22 very wide complexes per minute. The wide complexes come early and are not preceded by a P wave. What do you think has happened to G.S.? ❍ ❍ ❍ ❍ ❍

12. What should your next actions be?

13. What are the most likely causes of the abnormal beats?

14. You notice that G.S. looks frightened and is lying stiff as a board. How would you respond to this situation?

G.S.'s PVCs responded well to treatment. Unfortunately one week later, a large embolus lodged in her lungs. All attempts at resuscitation failed.

Case Study 13

Name ______________________ Class/Group ______ Date ______

Group Members ______________________________

INSTRUCTIONS: All questions apply to this case study. Your responses should be brief and to the point. Adequate space has been provided for answers. When asked to provide several answers, they should be listed in order of priority or significance. Do not assume information that is not provided. Please print or write clearly. If your response is not legible, it will be marked as ? and you will need to rewrite it.

❍ ❍ ❍ / ❍ ❍

Scenario

P.R., a 31-year-old woman diagnosed with Guillain-Barré syndrome, is being cared for on a special ventilator unit of an extended-care facility because she requires 24-hour/day nursing coverage. She has been intubated and mechanically ventilated for 3 weeks and has shown no signs of improvement in respiratory muscle strength. Her ventilator settings are A/C of 12, VT 700, FiO_2 .50, PEEP 5. Her VS are 108/64, 118, 12, 100.6° F. She is receiving enteral nutrition by nasal-duodenal tube (2800 calories/24 hours). P.R.'s three children, ages 3, 4, and 6, are staying with her sister, because he husband has to keep working his full-time job to maintain their medical insurance.

1. Why is P.R.'s ventilator mode on assist-control? ❍ ❍ ❍ ❍ ❍

2. P.R. is receiving lorazepam (Ativan) 1 mg slow IVP q4h to reduce her anxiety. Identify two factors that should be considered when choosing Ativan for P.R. ❍ ❍ ❍ ❍ ❍

3. Identify nine nonpharmacologic strategies that you could use to reduce P.R.'s anxiety, increase her comfort, and reduce the need for Ativan. Be creative! ❍ ❍ ❍ ❍ ❍

4. You give P.R. a bath and note that her cheeks billow outward each time the ventilator delivers a breath. What could cause this phenomenon?

5. You try repositioning P.R., place a stopcock in the inflation valve, auscultate the lungs, check the length of the tube at the lip (the tube had not moved), and finally insert more air in the cuff before sealing the leak. Over the next 24 hours, the leak becomes worse and the ventilator's low exhaled volume alarm repeatedly sounds. What action should you take?

6. The physician elects to insert a No. 8 Shiley tracheostomy tube with a disposable inner cannula. P.R. becomes increasingly anxious after receiving the news. How would you prepare P.R. and her husband for the tracheostomy?

7. P.R. undergoes the tracheostomy procedure without complications. When you return in the morning and assess the new tracheostomy, you note that the trach tape looks tight. You are unable to insert 1 finger between P.R.'s neck and the trach tape. Discuss whether or not this is problematic.

8. What should your next actions be?

9. You note that the tissue surrounding the incision is edematous. As you palpate the area, your fingers sink into the skin and you auscultate a popping sound through your stethoscope. Is this to be expected?

10. Based on your decision in question 9, what action should you take?

11. That afternoon, a powerful storm causes a power failure. What should you do?

12. Within minutes of the power failure, the rescue unit arrives at the door. How did they know you needed assistance?

13. You evaluate P.R.'s activity tolerance and note that she desaturates when turned to her R side. You auscultate tubular breath sounds in the entire R lung posteriorally. Based on your knowledge of pathophysiology, explain the probable cause of the desaturation.

You notify the physician of the change in P.R.'s breath sounds. The paramedic unit transports P.R. to the hospital, where she is readmitted for recurring pneumonia.

14. P.R.'s husband arrives shortly after the paramedics transport P.R. to the hospital. He collapses into the nearest chair, tears begin to roll down his cheeks, and he says, "It has been almost a month now. Are you sure she will recover?" How would you respond?

P.R. undergoes aggressive antibiotic therapy and is discharged to home 5 days later. She progresses slowly. It takes nearly a year for her to recover, but recovery is complete.

Case Study 14

Name ______________________ Class/Group ______ Date ______

Group Members ______________________________________

INSTRUCTIONS: All questions apply to this case study. Your responses should be brief and to the point. Adequate space has been provided for answers. When asked to provide several answers, they should be listed in order of priority or significance. Do not assume information that is not provided. Please print or write clearly. If your response is not legible, it will be marked as ? and you will need to rewrite it.

Scenario

D.Z., a 65-year-old man, is admitted to a medical floor for exacerbation of his emphysema (COPD). He has a PMH of HTN, which has been well controlled by enalopril for the last six years. He presents as a thin, poorly nourished man who is experiencing difficulty breathing. He c/o coughing spells that are productive of thick yellow sputum. D.Z. seems irritable and anxious when he tells you that he has been a 2-pack-a-day smoker for 38 years. He c/o sleeping poorly and lately feels very tired most of the time. His VS are 162/84, 124, 36, 102° F, SaO_2 88%. His admitting diagnosis is chronic emphysema with an acute exacerbation; etiology to be determined. His admitting orders are as follows: diet as tolerated; out of bed with assistance; O_2 at 2 L/NC; maintenance IV of D_5W at 50 ml/h; sputum C&S x 3; ABGs in AM; hemogram with diff., basic metabolic panel, and theophylline level on admission; CXR in AM; prednisone 40 mg PO tid; cefuroxime 1 g IVPB q8h and azithromycin 2 g IVPB q8h; theophylline (Theo-Dur) 300 mg PO bid; albuterol 2.5 mg (0.5 ml) in 3 ml NS q6h and ipatropium 500 mcg (unit-dose vial), both by oral nebulization; enalapril (Vasotec) 10 mg PO q AM.

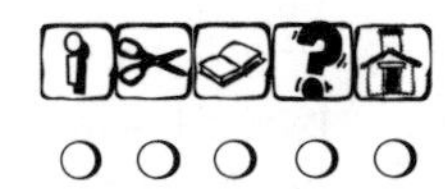

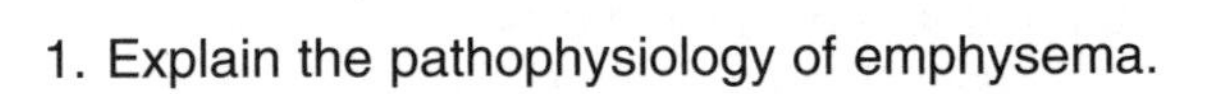

1. Explain the pathophysiology of emphysema.

2. Are D.Z.'s VS and SaO_2 appropriate? If not, explain why.

3. Identify three nursing measures you could try to improve oxygenation.

4. Explain the main purpose of the following classes of drugs: antibiotics, bronchodilators, and corticosteroids.

5. What are the two most common side effects of bronchodilators?

6. You deliver D.Z.'s dietary tray, and he comments how hungry he is. As you leave the room, he is rapidly consuming the mashed potatoes. When you pick up the tray, you notice that he hasn't touched anything else. When you question him, he states, "I don't understand it. I can be so hungry, but when I start to eat, I have trouble breathing and I have to stop." Explain this phenomenon based on your knowledge of the breakdown of carbohydrates (CHO).

7. Identify four strategies that might improve his caloric intake.

8. Identify three expected outcomes of D.Z.'s treatment.

9. You answer D.Z.'s call light, and he asks for a carton of milk. You remind him that milk causes an increased production of thick mucus. He replies, "Yes, but you told me that I need lots of protein." How should you respond?

10. You notice a box of dark chocolate on D.Z.'s overbed table. He tells you that he wakes at night and eats four or five pieces of chocolate. Several of your COPD patients have identified a craving for chocolate in the past. What is the basis for this craving?

11. What would you do to address dietary and nutritional teaching needs with D.Z. and his wife?

12. List six educational topics that you need to explore with D.Z.

13. What other health care professional would probably be involved in D.Z.'s treatments and how? What is the licensure/certification status of that profession in the state in which you are practicing?

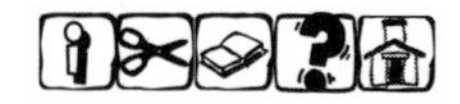

D.Z.'s wife approaches you in the hallway and says, "I don't know what to do. My husband used to be so active before he retired 6 months ago. Since then, he's lost 35 pounds. He is afraid to take a bath and it takes him hours to dress—that's if he gets dressed at all. He has gone downhill so fast that it scares me. He's afraid to do anything for himself. He wants me in the room with him all the time, but if I try to talk with him, he snarls and does things to irritate me. I have to keep working. His medical bills are draining all our savings, and I have to be able to support myself when he's gone. You know, sometimes I go to work just to get away from the house and his constant demands. He calls me several times a day asking me to come home, but I can't go home. You may not think I'm much of a wife, but quite honestly, I don't want to come home anymore. I just don't know what to do."

14. How would you respond to her? ❍ ❍ ❍ ❍ ❍

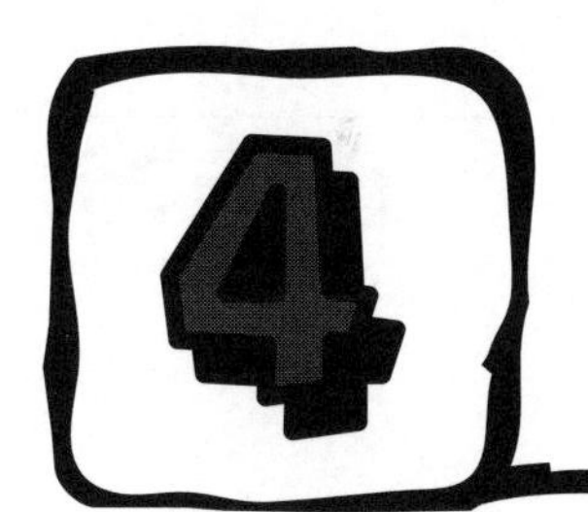

Musculoskeletal Disorders

Case Study 1

Name ______________________ Class/Group ______ Date ______

Group Members ____

INSTRUCTIONS: All questions apply to this case study. Your responses should be brief and to the point. Adequate space has been provided for answers. When asked to provide several answers, they should be listed in order of priority or significance. Do not assume information that is not provided. Please print or write clearly. If your response is not legible, it will be marked as ? and you will need to rewrite it.

Scenario

M.B. is a 55-year-old woman presenting to the clinic with c/o episodes of feeling "hot and sweaty" during the day and waking up at night soaked with perspiration. Because her sleep is so disrupted, she is tired all day and is having trouble concentrating at work. She says that the episodes are becoming unbearable and is seeking treatment for them.

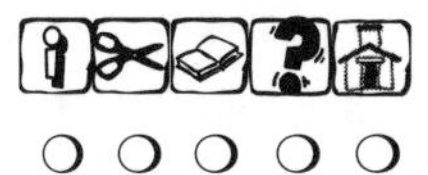

1. You suspect M.B. is perimenopausal. You obtain her prior medical and surgical history and her current medication regimen. List three questions that would be important to ask in exploring the possibility of menopause being r/t her symptoms.

2. You are concerned with the possible development of osteoporosis in M.B. List at least eight questions you would ask to determine her risk for development of osteoporosis.

3. M.B. is not currently taking estrogen replacement therapy. What three questions would be important to ask M.B. to determine whether there are any contraindications or precautions to this therapy for her?

4. M.B. says that she does have frequent "backaches." Spinal films (x-rays) are ordered. Later you see a report stating that the films appear normal with no significant findings. What would be an appropriate explanation of these findings?

5. What would be appropriate supportive measures for M.B. to relieve the noninjury-related low back pain in the absence of fracture? ❍ ❍ ❍ ❍ ❍

6. M.B. reports that she does not like milk or milk products and rarely includes them in her diet. How can M.B. increase her calcium intake at this time? ❍ ❍ ❍ ❍ ❍

7. M.B.'s physician told her that her blood calcium was normal. "If I have enough calcium in my blood, I couldn't have osteoporosis, could I?" she asks you. How will you respond and why? ❍ ❍ ❍ ❍ ❍

8. M.B. says she rarely exercises. What advice should be given concerning exercise? ❍ ❍ ❍ ❍ ❍

9. M.S. states she still is not certain she has a well-balanced diet with sufficient calcium and vitamin D. What would you suggest to her? ❍ ❍ ❍ ❍ ❍

Back to her CC, "hot flashes": M.S. was given a prescription for 0.625 mg Premarin. Look it up—what are the indications (reasons it would be prescribed) and contraindications? Note why it would be useful for someone with hot flashes.

10. What side effects may be experienced with Premarin and what instructions should be given someone receiving it?

Note: A recent scientific study found that one-third of the individuals in a group who had an MI suffered no chest pain at all.

Note: A lot of osteoporosis in older women, as well as men, develops as secondary to gastric problems, renal disorders, arthritis, and medication intake. Also, deficits in calcium intake is relatively common among low-income people with poor nutrition or in elderly individuals living alone.

Case Study 2

Name ________________________ Class/Group ______ Date ______

Group Members ____

INSTRUCTIONS: All questions apply to this case study. Your responses should be brief and to the point. Adequate space has been provided for answers. When asked to provide several answers, they should be listed in order of priority or significance. Do not assume information that is not provided. Please print or write clearly. If your response is not legible, it will be marked as ? and you will need to rewrite it.

❍ ❍ ❍ / ❍ ❍

Scenario

J.C. is a 41-year-old man who comes to the ED c/o acute low back pain. He states that he did some heavy lifting yesterday, went to bed with a mild backache, and awoke this morning with terrible back pain. He admits to having had several episodes of similar back pain each year over the last 10 years. In the past, the pain has been treated by diazepam, codeine, NSAIDs, and several weeks of bed rest. J.C. had a PMH of a peptic ulcer. He is 6 ft tall, weighs 265 lb, and has a prominent "pot belly." The ED admitting clerk calls J.C.'s insurance company to authorize payment for treatment at your facility. J.C.'s HMO has identified him as a consumer of "high-cost care" with poor prior outcome. The ED is authorized to perform emergency treatment only and the case manager will make a home visit within 24 hours to devise a treatment plan. The ED physician diagnoses muscular strain of the lower back and orders the following: cyclobenzaprene (Flexeril) 10 mg QID, Celebrex 200 mg QD; bed rest for 2 days then gradually increase activity; ice packs to the lower back 30 minutes out of every hour.

You are a case manager (RN) working for Grubabuck HMO and make the initial visit to J.C.'s residence. His wife lets you in and you find J.C. lying on the sofa with his knees flexed and watching videos.

1. What questions would be appropriate to ask J.C. in evaluating the extent of his back pain and injury? ❍ ❍ ❍ ❍ ❍

2. What observable characteristic does J.C. have that makes him highly susceptible to low back injury and chronic pain? ❍ ❍ ❍ ❍ ❍

3. Why do you think that cyclobenzaprine was prescribed instead of diazepam? ❍ ❍ ❍ ❍ ❍

4. J.C. used to take piroxicam 20 mg until he developed his duodonal ulcer. What is the relationship between the two? What s/s would you expect if an ulcer developed? ❍ ❍ ❍ ❍ ❍

You determine that J.C. needs an interdisciplinary approach to treatment and rehabilitation for his chronic back problem. Your goal is to minimize J.C.'s long-term health care costs by rehabilitating his back, helping him reduce his weight to reduce stress on his back, and treating his current injury. You coordinate referrals for J.C. to see four health care experts on your team.

5. You refer J.C. to a physiatrist. What is a physiatrist, and what can a physiatrist do to help J.C.? ❍ ❍ ❍ ❍ ❍

6. What expert would work with J.C. to help him lose weight? What are this expert's credentials? ❍ ❍ ❍ ❍ ❍

7. What kind of expert will work with J.C. using exercise and various treatment modalities to restore his back muscles? ❍ ❍ ❍ ❍ ❍

8. What kind of expert will work with J.C. on body mechanics and strengthening him for occupational- and home-related work? ❍ ❍ ❍ ❍ ❍

9. A PT teaches J.C. maintenance exercises he can do on his own to promote back health. What 3 common exercises would be included?

10. What is Celebrex, and how does it work? Name at least one other drug in the same drug family. What advantage do these medications have over the "older" NSAIDs?

11. Why would you want to use an NSAID rather than acetaminophen for pain?

Case Study 3

Name ______________________ Class/Group ______ Date ______

Group Members ____

INSTRUCTIONS: All questions apply to this case study. Your responses should be brief and to the point. Adequate space has been provided for answers. When asked to provide several answers, they should be listed in order of priority or significance. Do not assume information that is not provided. Please print or write clearly. If your response is not legible, it will be marked as ? and you will need to rewrite it.

Scenario

D.M., a 25-year-old man, hops into the ED c/o right ankle pain. He states that he was playing basketball and stepped on another player's foot, inverting his ankle. You note swelling over the lateral malleolus down to the area of the fourth and fifth metatarsal, and pedal pulses are 3+ bilaterally. His VS are 124/76, 82, 18. He has no allergies and takes no medication. He states he has had no prior surgeries or medical problems.

1. When assessing D.M.'s injured ankle, what should be evaluated?

2. What should initial nursing management of the ankle involve to prevent further swelling and injury to the ankle?

3. You note there is significant swelling over the fourth and fifth metatarsal. How would you further evaluate this finding?

X-rays are negative for fracture, and a third-degree sprain is diagnosed. The physician orders an ankle splint with elastic wrap and crutches with instructions. The physician instructs D.M. not to bear weight on his ankle for 2 days.

4. Describe the technique for applying an elastic wrap. Give the rationale.

5. When instructing D.M. to use crutches, his weight should rest on what part of his body while the crutch is bearing the weight? Explain why.

6. You are to instruct D.M. on application of cold and heat, activity, and care of the ankle. What would be appropriate instructions in these areas?

7. D.M. is given a prescription for acetominophen/hydrocodone (Lortab) for pain. What instructions concerning this medication should you give him on discharge?

8. Four days later D.M. hobbles into the ED and boldly informs you that he "did it again, only this time it was touch football." He states that the pain pills worked so well, he thought it would be OK. You detect the odor of beer on his breath. What are you going to do?

9. You remove his sock and find a large hematoma forming on the lateral aspect of an already-swollen ankle. The ankle also shows the color of a bruise that is several days old. You inquire about D.M.'s pain perception. He states, "It doesn't feel too bad now, but I sure saw stars when it popped." What is the significance of his statement?

Case Study 4

Name ______________________ Class/Group ______ Date ______

Group Members ______________________________________

INSTRUCTIONS: All questions apply to this case study. Your responses should be brief and to the point. Adequate space has been provided for answers. When asked to provide several answers, they should be listed in order of priority or significance. Do not assume information that is not provided. Please print or write clearly. If your response is not legible, it will be marked as ? and you will need to rewrite it.

❍ ❍ ❍ / ❍ ❍

Scenario

S.P. is admitted to the orthopedic ward. She has fallen at home and has sustained an intracapsular fracture of the hip at the femoral neck. The following history is obtained from her: She is a 75-year-old widow with 3 children living nearby. Her father died of cancer at 62 years of age; mother died of CHF at 79 years of age. Ht 5'3", wt 118 lb. She has a 50 pack-year smoking history and denies alcohol use. She had severe rheumatoid arthritis with UGI bleed in 1993 and CAD with CABG 9 months ago. Since that time she has engaged in "very mild exercises at home." VS are 128/60, 98, 14, 37.2° C. Medications: nizatidine (Axid) 150 mg bid, prednisone (Deltasone) 5 mg PO qd, and methotrexate (Amethopterin) 2.5 mg/weekly.

1. List four risk factors for hip fractures. ❍ ❍ ❍ ❍ ❍

2. Place a check mark next to each of the responses in question 1 that represent S.P.'s risk factors. ❍ ❍ ❍ ❍ ❍

S.P. is taken to surgery for a total hip replacement. Because of the intracapsular location of the fracture, the surgeon chooses to perform an arthroplasty rather than internal fixation.

3. What is the difference between arthroplasty and open reduction and internal fixation (ORIF)? ❍ ❍ ❍ ❍ ❍

4. List four critical potential postoperative problems for S.P., and explain why you think each is important.

5. How would you monitor for excessive postoperative blood loss?

6. There are two main goals for maintaining proper alignment of S.P.'s operative leg. What are they, and how are they achieved?

7. Postoperative wound infection is a concern for S.P. Describe what you would do to monitor S.P. for wound infection.

8. Taking S.P's rheumatoid arthritis into consideration, what interventions should be implemented to prevent complications secondary to immobility?

9. What predisposing factor, identified in S.P.'s medical history, places her at risk for infection, bleeding, and anemia?

10. Briefly discuss S.P.'s nutritional needs.

11. Explain four techniques you can teach S.P. to help her protect herself from infection r/t medication-induced immune suppression.

S.P. was transferred to a long-term care facility for rehabilitation.

Case Study 5

Name ______________________ Class/Group ______ Date ______

Group Members ______________________________

INSTRUCTIONS: All questions apply to this case study. Your responses should be brief and to the point. Adequate space has been provided for answers. When asked to provide several answers, they should be listed in order of priority or significance. Do not assume information that is not provided. Please print or write clearly. If your response is not legible, it will be marked as ? and you will need to rewrite it.

Scenario

H.K. is a 26-year-old man who tried to light a cigarette while driving and lost control of his Jeep. The Jeep flipped and landed on the passenger side. H.K. was transported to the ED with a deformed, edematous R lower leg and a deep puncture wound approximately 5 cm long over the deformity. Blood continues to ooze from the wound.

1. What further assessment should the nurse make of the leg injury and what precautions should she take in making this assessment?

2. What would be the most appropriate method for controlling bleeding at this wound site?

3. From the above information, it is clear that H.K. is a smoker. List at least three issues r/t his smoking that can complicate his care and recovery. What nursing interventions could be instituted to counter these complications? Would using a nicotine patch eliminate these problems?

4. What is the best way to immobilize the leg injury prior to surgery?

H.K. is taken to surgery for ORIF of the tibia and fibula fractures. He returns with a full leg fiberglass cast with windows over the areas of surgery.

5. Describe nursing assessment of a patient with a long leg cast involving trauma and surgery.

6. In assessing H.K.'s cast on the third day postop, you notice a strong foul odor. Drainage on the cast is extending, and H.K. is c/o pain more often and seems considerably more uncomfortable. VS are 123/78, 102, 18, 39° C. What is your analysis of these findings?

H.K. returns to surgery. The wound over H.K.'s fracture site has become necrotic with purulent drainage. The wound is debrided and cultured; then a posterior splint is applied. H.K. returns to his room with orders for wet-to-moist dressing changes. The physician suspects osteomyelitis and orders nafcillin (Unipen), and gentamycin (Gentak).

7. As you continue to assess H.K. over the following days, what evidence will you look for that antibiotics are effectively treating the infection?

8. What should H.K. be taught concerning the care of his cast?

9. What nutritional needs will H.K. have, and why?

10. To ensure pain management, H.K. is given a 75 mcg transdermal fentanyl patch. What therapeutic category does this drug belong to? What s/s would you see if he were to have a toxic or overdose reaction?

11. What is the antidote to toxic narcotic reactions, and how is it administered?

Case Study 6

Name ____________________ Class/Group ______ Date ______

Group Members ____________________

INSTRUCTIONS: All questions apply to this case study. Your responses should be brief and to the point. Adequate space has been provided for answers. When asked to provide several answers, they should be listed in order of priority or significance. Do not assume information that is not provided. Please print or write clearly. If your response is not legible, it will be marked as ? and you will need to rewrite it.

❍ ❍ ❍ / ❍ ❍

Scenario

M.M., a 76-year-old retired schoolteacher, underwent ORIF of his R femur. He has been on bed rest for the first 2 days postoperatively. 0600 VS were 132/84, 80 reg, 18 unlabored, and 37.2° C. He is AA&O (awake, alert, and oriented). No adventitious heart sounds. Breath sounds are clear but diminished in the bases bilaterally. Bowel sounds are present, and he is taking sips of clear liquids. An IV of $D_5 \frac{1}{2}$NS is infusing TKO in his L hand and should be saline locked in the AM if he is able to maintain adequate PO fluid intake. His lab work shows Hct 34%, Hgb 11.3 mg/dL, K 4.1 mmol/L, PTT 44 seconds. Pain is controlled with morphine sulfate 4 mg IV and promethazine (Phenergan) 25 mg IV q3h. He is also taking Nitropatch, heparin 5000 units SQ bid, and docusate sodium.

At 2330 on the second postoperative day, you answer M.M.'s call light and find him lying in bed breathing rapidly and rubbing his R chest. He is c/o R-sided chest pain and appears to be restless.

1. What are you going to do? ❍ ❍ ❍ ❍ ❍

He is slightly hypotensive, tachycardic, tachypneic, restless, and slightly confused. The pulse oximeter reads 86%, so you start him on 3–6 L O_2/nc. You identify faint crackles in the posterior bases bilaterally; they were clear this AM.

2. Based on your findings, you call the physician. What information are you going to give him? ❍ ❍ ❍ ❍ ❍

3. The physician orders ABGs on room air, continuous pulse oximetry, STAT CXR, and STAT 12-lead ECG. What information will the physician gain from each of the above?

4. Why would the physician order ABGs on room air as opposed to with supplemental O_2?

The ABGs return as follows: pH 7.55, $PaCO_2$ 24 mmHg, HCO_3 24 mmol/L, and PaO_2 56 mmHg at sea level. SaO_2 is 86% on room air. Chest x-ray shows a small R infiltrate. VS are 150/92, 110, 28, 37.2° C.

5. What is your interpretation of the ABGs, and what do you think the physician will order next?

6. The V/Q is performed, and the interpretation reads "strongly suggestive of a pulmonary embolus." What are the most likely sources of the embolus?

7. Based on the latest PTT of 40 seconds, the physician orders a heparin bolus of 5000 units IV followed by an infusion of 1200 units/hour. Based on these results, what action would you take?

The PTT 4 hours later is >120 seconds.

8. The next day, the physician's orders read, "Coumadin 2.5 mg, PT/INR in AM, DC heparin." What is wrong with these orders?

9. Thrombolytics, such as streptokinase and urokinase, have been beneficial in the treatment of pulmonary embolus. Why would this medication be contraindicated in M.M.'s case?

10. List three priority nursing problems r/t the care of M.M. in his current situation.

11. Several days later, you hear M.M. requesting his son to bring in a "decent razor" because he is tired of the stubble left by the unit's shaver. How would you address this issue?

Case Study 7

Name ____________________ Class/Group ______ Date ______

Group Members ____________________

INSTRUCTIONS: All questions apply to this case study. Your responses should be brief and to the point. Adequate space has been provided for answers. When asked to provide several answers, they should be listed in order of priority or significance. Do not assume information that is not provided. Please print or write clearly. If your response is not legible, it will be marked as ? and you will need to rewrite it.

Scenario

You are working in the ED when a 27-year-old man runs through the door with a blood-soaked towel over his left hand. D.W., a machinist, states he caught his hand in an automatic shear and cut off his left index finger. His coworker has the finger wrapped in a paper towel. You grab a pair of gloves while you direct D.W. to lie on a stretcher where you remove the towel and apply firm pressure to the stump with sterile sponges. Another nurse takes his VS and announces 196/122, 144, 22. To distract him, you gather information about his PMH, allergies, and tetanus status. He has a history of depression, for which he takes Prozac, and he is allergic to Darvocet. He has no significant medical history other than depression.

1. What is your first nursing priority in dealing with D.W.'s amputated finger?

2. D.W.'s stump is bleeding profusely. Would you apply a tourniquet to the end of the finger or not, and why?

3. An x-ray of the index finger reveals an amputation of the proximal DIP joint. The fracture has left a jagged protruding bone that can be seen from the distal tip. After controlling the bleeding, what would be the appropriate management?

Note: Observe D.W.'s anxiety level and LOC, and assess for shock. Make sure he is in a stable condition in case he goes into shock and/or loses consciousness.

4. What would be suitable treatment of the amputated appendage?

5. D.W. has not had a tetanus shot in the last 10 years. You have run out of adult TD and you only have pediatric DPT available. Would it be suitable to give the pediatric DPT?

6. What factors influence the success of the reattached digit?

7. List three issues related to D.W.'s care.

8. You repeat his VS and record the following: 118/86, 78, 18. Do you find the VS changes to be reassuring or distressing, and why?

9. The OR calls for D.M. Before he leaves, you need to start an IV. What type of solution would you hang, and why?

10. Why would it be important to further question D.M. about his allergy to Darvocet?

D.M. was prescribed 1–2 Percocet q4–6h prn for pain.

Case Study 8

Name ______________________ Class/Group ______ Date ______

Group Members ____

INSTRUCTIONS: All questions apply to this case study. Your responses should be brief and to the point. Adequate space has been provided for answers. When asked to provide several answers, they should be listed in order of priority or significance. Do not assume information that is not provided. Please print or write clearly. If your response is not legible, it will be marked as ? and you will need to rewrite it.

Scenario

B.G. is struck by a vehicle while riding his motorcycle and is transported to your ED by ambulance. He is found to have a fractured mandible and multiple fractures of the R tibia and fibula.

1. When a patient comes in with facial trauma such as B.G.'s, what two other injuries should you assume exist until ruled out? Explain.

B.G. is taken to the OR for intermaxillary fixation (wiring of the jaw) and pinning of the fractured tibia and fibula.

2. B.G. returns from surgery with his jaws wired. What patient care issue r/t his wired jaws would you be concerned about postoperatively?

HINT: Think in terms of an emergency.

3. What precautions will you take to ensure a patent airway in B.G. if he begins vomiting while his jaws are wired?

4. If B.G. begins vomiting with his jaws wired, what actions should you take?

B.C. is transferred to a rehabilitation facility for treatment of his leg injury.

5. His jaw remains wired. What instructions should you give him concerning oral care and safety?

6. During his stay at the rehabilitation facility, what nutritional teaching does B.G. need to prepare him for discharge?

B.G. has daily dressing changes, antibiotics, and PT; wound debridement is prn.

7. Two weeks after B.G.'s accident, you enter his room to do his afternoon shift assessment. The shades are drawn, he is sitting in the corner with his face to the wall, and you have been told he refused to go to PT this afternoon. He answers your questions in flat, monosyllabic tones. When you ask him what is wrong, he explodes in anger, even more frustrated because his wired jaw keeps him from being able to talk well. What are you going to do?

8. B.G. tells you, "I got a good look at my leg today when the bandage was off. It looks really ugly. I wanted to throw up." What are you going to say? ❍ ❍ ❍ ❍ ❍

B.G. was discharged to home but returned to the rehabilitation facility for PT and continued wound management for 3 months. Several months later you see B.G. at the grocery store. You call his name; he waves and walks toward you. You notice that he walks with a slight limp. He tells you that his leg healed, but he has pain in his knee when he walks or hikes any distance.

9. What could be causing pain in B.G.'s R knee? (Remember that his R foreleg had originally been injured.) ❍ ❍ ❍ ❍ ❍

10. You suggest B.G. ask his physician about a prescription for a foot evaluation and orthotics. What are orthotics, and what purpose do they serve? ❍ ❍ ❍ ❍ ❍

B.G. will be referred to a sports medicine center, orthopedist, podiatrist, or PT to have his gait and foot evaluated.

Case Study 9

Name ______________________ Class/Group ______ Date ______

Group Members ____________________________________

INSTRUCTIONS: All questions apply to this case study. Your responses should be brief and to the point. Adequate space has been provided for answers. When asked to provide several answers, they should be listed in order of priority or significance. Do not assume information that is not provided. Please print or write clearly. If your response is not legible, it will be marked as ? and you will need to rewrite it.

Scenario

J.F., a 67-year-old woman, was involved in an auto accident and is life-flighted to your facility. She sustained a ruptured spleen, fractured pelvis, and compound fractures of the L femur. On admission she underwent a splenectomy (5 days ago). Her pelvis was stabilized with an external fixator device 3 days ago, and yesterday her L femur was stabilized using balanced suspension with skeletal traction. She has a Thomas ring with Pearson attachment on her L leg. She has 20 lb of skeletal traction and 5 lb applied to the balanced suspension. Her L femur is elevated off the bed at approximately 45 degrees. The foreleg (lower part of her leg) is parallel to the bed and lies in a sling that the nurse adjusts on the frame, and the foot hangs freely. This morning J.F. was transferred to your orthopedic unit for specialized care. You are the nurse assigned to care for her on the night shift.

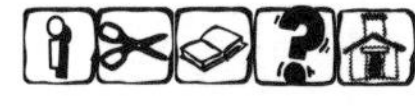

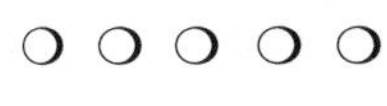

1. You enter J.F.'s room for the first time. What aspects of the traction would you want to inspect?

2. When inspecting the skeletal pin sites, you note that the skin is reddened for an inch around the pin on both the medial and lateral L leg. What does this finding indicate, and what action would you take?

3. You find J.F.'s body in the lower 75% of the bed, her L upper leg at an exaggerated angle (>45 degrees.) The knot at the end of the bed is caught in the pulley, and the 20-lb weight is dangling just above the floor. What are you going to do?

4. When you lift J.F., you notice that her sheets are wet. Because you have lots of help in the room, you decide to change J.F.'s linen. How would you accomplish this task?

5. J.F. tells you that she feels like she needs to have a bowel movement, but it is too painful to sit on the bedpan. How would you respond?

6. J.F. expels a few small, hard, round pieces of stool. What could be done to promote normal elimination?

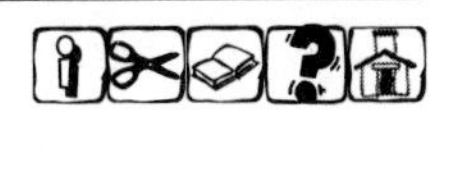

You ask J.F. if she is ready for her bath, and she responds positively. You let her bathe the parts she can reach and engage her in a conversation as you attend to the rest of her body. While performing peri care you notice that the folds of skin around her peri area are reddened and excoriated.

7. Given that J.F. has been on antibiotics for the last 5 days, what is the likely cause of the problem, and what needs to be done to encourage healing? ❍ ❍ ❍ ❍ ❍

8. You ask J.F. what she is doing to exercise while she is confined to bed. She looks surprised and states that she isn't doing anything. What activities can J.F. engage in while on bed rest? ❍ ❍ ❍ ❍ ❍

9. You realize that maintaining skin integrity is a challenge in J.F.'s case. What measures will you take to prevent skin breakdown? ❍ ❍ ❍ ❍ ❍

10. Although J.F. is recovering nicely, she is becoming increasingly withdrawn. You enter her room and find her crying. She tells you that she is all alone here, that she misses her family terribly. You know that her son is flying into town tomorrow but will only be able to stay a few days. What can be done so that J.F. benefits from her family support system? ❍ ❍ ❍ ❍ ❍

Case Study 10

Name ______________________ Class/Group ______ Date ______

Group Members ____

INSTRUCTIONS: All questions apply to this case study. Your responses should be brief and to the point. Adequate space has been provided for answers. When asked to provide several answers, they should be listed in order of priority or significance. Do not assume information that is not provided. Please print or write clearly. If your response is not legible, it will be marked as ? and you will need to rewrite it.

Scenario

You are working in the ED when M.C., an 82-year-old widow, arrives by ambulance. Because M.C. had not answered her phone since noon yesterday, her daughter went to her home to check on her. She found M.C. lying on the kitchen floor, incontinent of urine and stool, and c/o pain in her R hip. Her daughter reports a PMH of hypertension, angina, and osteoporosis. M.C. takes propanolol (Inderal), nitropatch, indapamide (Lozol), and Premarin daily. The daughter reports that her mother is normally very alert and lives independently. Upon examination, you see an elderly woman, approximately 100 lb, holding her right thigh. You note shortening of the right leg with external rotation and a large amount of swelling at the proximal thigh and right hip. M.C. is oriented to person only and is confused about place and time. M.C.'s VS are 90/65, 120, 24, 36.4° C; her SaO_2 is 89%. She is profoundly dehydrated. Preliminary diagnosis is fracture of the right hip.

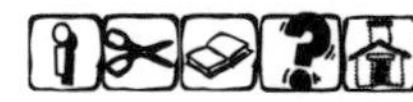

1. In view of M.C.'s history of hypertension and the fact that she has been without her medications for at least 24 hours, explain her current VS.

2. Based on her history and your initial assessment, what three priority interventions should be initiated?

3. M.C.'s daughter states, "Mother is always so clear and alert. I have never seen her act so confused. What's wrong with her?" What are 3 possible causes for M.C.'s disorientation that should be considered and evaluated?

X-ray films confirmed the diagnosis of intertrochanteric femoral fracture. Knowing that M.C. is going to be admitted, you draw admission labs and call for an orthopedic consult.

4. What laboratory and diagnostic studies would be ordered to evaluate M.C.'s condition, and what critical information will each give you?

5. What are the 5 Ps that should guide the assessment of M.C.'s right leg before and after surgery?

6. In evaluating M.C.'s pulses, you find her posterior tibial pulse and dorsalis pedis pulse to be weaker on her right foot than on her left. What would be a possible cause of this finding?

7. In planning further care for M.C., list four potential complications for which M.C. should be monitored.

8. M.C. keeps asking about "Peaches." No one seems to be paying attention. You ask her what she means. She says Peaches is her little dog and she's worried about who is taking care of her. How will you answer?

❍ ❍ ❍ ❍ ❍

M.C. is placed in Buck's traction and sent to the orthopedic unit until an ORIF can be scheduled. Lortab is ordered for severe pain with orders for acetaminophen and Ultram for mild and moderate pain, respectively. M.C.'s cardiovascular, pulmonary, and renal status are closely monitored.

9. Ultram and Lortab are narcotics and therefore constipating. What would you do to prevent constipation?

❍ ❍ ❍ ❍ ❍

10. What is obstipation?

❍ ❍ ❍ ❍ ❍

After her surgery, M.C. is transferred to a long-term care facility for PT/OT rehabilitation. She is placed on prophylactic Coumadin.

Case Study 11

Name ______________________ Class/Group ______ Date ______

Group Members ____

INSTRUCTIONS: All questions apply to this case study. Your responses should be brief and to the point. Adequate space has been provided for answers. When asked to provide several answers, they should be listed in order of priority or significance. Do not assume information that is not provided. Please print or write clearly. If your response is not legible, it will be marked as ? and you will need to rewrite it.

❍ ❍ ❍ / ❍ ❍

Scenario

E.B., a 69-year-old man with type 1 diabetes mellitus (DM), is admitted to a large, regional medical center c/o severe pain in his R foot and lower leg. The foot and lower leg are cool and without pulses (absent by Doppler). Arteriogram demonstrates severe atherosclerosis of the right popliteal artery with complete obstruction of blood flow. Despite attempts at endarterectomy and intravascular urokinase over several days, the foot and lower leg become necrotic. Finally, the decision is made to perform an AKA (above-the-knee amputation) on E.B.'s R leg. E.B. is recently widowed and has a son and daughter who live nearby. In preparation for E.B.'s surgery, the surgeons wish to spare as much viable tissue as possible. Hence an order is written for E.B. to undergo 5 days of hyperbaric therapy for 20 minutes bid.

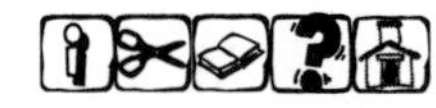

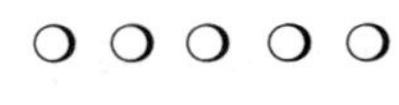

1. What is the purpose of hyperbaric therapy, and what purpose does it serve in a patient like E.B.?

As you are preparing E.B. for surgery, he is quiet and withdrawn. He follows instructions quietly and slowly without asking questions. His son and daughter are at his bedside and they also are very quiet. Finally, E.B. says, "I don't want to go like your mother did. She lingered on and had so much pain. I don't want them to bring me back."

2. You look at his chart and find no advance directives. What is your responsibility? ❍ ❍ ❍ ❍ ❍

3. What is your assessment of E.B.'s behavior at this time? ❍ ❍ ❍ ❍ ❍

4. What are some appropriate nursing interventions and responses to E.B.'s anticipatory grief? ❍ ❍ ❍ ❍ ❍

E.B. returns from surgery with the right stump dressed with gauze and an elastic wrap. The dressing is dry and intact, without drainage. He is drowsy with the following VS: 142/80, 96, 14, 36.6° C. He has a maintenance IV of D_5.9NS infusing at 125 ml/h in his right forearm.

5. The surgeon has written to keep E.B.'s stump elevated on pillows for 48 hours; after that, have him lay in prone position for 15 minutes qid. In teaching E.B. about his care, how would you explain the rationale for these orders? ❍ ❍ ❍ ❍ ❍

6. In reviewing E.B.'s medical history, what factor may affect the condition of his stump and ultimate rehabilitation potential? ❍ ❍ ❍ ❍ ❍

You have just returned from a 2-day workshop on guidelines for the care of surgical patients with type 1 DM. You notice that E.B.'s blood glucose has been running between 130 to 180. The sliding scale insulin intervention does not begin until a blood glucose of 200 is reported. You recognize that patients with blood glucoses even slightly above normal suffer from impaired wound healing.

7. Identify four interventions that would facilitate timely healing of E.B.'s stump. ❍ ❍ ❍ ❍ ❍

8. What should the postoperative assessment of E.B.'s stump dressing include? ❍ ❍ ❍ ❍ ❍

9. On the evening of the first postop day, E.B. becomes more awake and begins to c/o pain. He states, "My leg is really hurting; are you sure it's gone?" How would you respond to E.B.'s question? ❍ ❍ ❍ ❍ ❍

E.B. will be discharged to an extended-care facility for strength training; once the patient receives his prosthesis, he will receive balance training. After that, he will be discharged to his daughter's home.

10. What instructions should be given to E.B.'s daughter concerning safety around the home at this time? ❍ ❍ ❍ ❍ ❍

Case Study 12

Name ______________________ Class/Group ______ Date ______

Group Members ____

INSTRUCTIONS: All questions apply to this case study. Your responses should be brief and to the point. Adequate space has been provided for answers. When asked to provide several answers, they should be listed in order of priority or significance. Do not assume information that is not provided. Please print or write clearly. If your response is not legible, it will be marked as ? and you will need to rewrite it.

❍ ❍ ❍ / ❍ ❍

Scenario

J.T. has injured his hand at work and is accompanied to the ED by a coworker. You examine his hand and find a piece of a drill bit sticking out of the skin between the third and fourth knuckle of his left hand. There is another puncture site about an inch below and toward the center of the hand. Bleeding is minimal. J.T. is 41 years old, has no significant medical history, and NKDA (no known drug allergies). He states the accident occurred when a mill at work malfunctioned and knocked his hand onto a rack of drill bits. His last tetanus booster was 3 years ago. It is your job to provide the initial care for J.T.'s injury.

1. You examine J.T.'s hand. What should you include in your initial assessment, and why? ❍ ❍ ❍ ❍ ❍

You record that J.T.'s fingers are warm with capillary refill <2 seconds. Sensory perception is intact. He is able to flex and extend the distal joints but not the proximal joints of the third and fourth fingers.

2. You notice J.T.'s wedding band and promptly ask him to remove it. Why is this important? ❍ ❍ ❍ ❍ ❍

3. J.T. asks you why he can't just pull the bit out and go home. How should you respond to his question?

4. What common diagnostic test will identify fractures and the location of metal fragments in J.T.'s hand?

The drill bit is impaled ½ inch below the surface of the skin, and there are no fractures. Because the hand contains so many blood vessels, nerves, ligaments and tendons, the ED physician decides to consult a surgical hand specialist. A neurologic consult says there is no nerve damage. The surgeon suspects tendon damage and decides to operate immediately.

5. What do you need to do to prepare J.T. for immediate surgery?

6. You record that J.T. has had no food "since 8:00 PM yesterday" and drank "some water" this AM. Based on this information, do you anticipate problems during surgery, and why?

7. Should J.T. be given a tetanus booster before he goes to surgery?

The surgeon repairs two partially severed tendons and wraps the hand in a very large, padded dressing. The distal ½ inch of each digit protrudes from the bulky dressing.

8. While in the short-stay recovery area, J.T. asks the nurse why his fingers look yellowish-brown. How should she respond to his question?

The surgeon tells J.T. that he had to repair tendons in his third and fourth fingers and instructs J.T. that he is not to work. He gives J.T. prescriptions for an antibiotic and an antiinflammatory agent. He instructs J.T. to make an appointment to see him in the surgery clinic in 2 days.

9. What instructions should the nurse in the short-stay area discuss with J.T. and his wife before releasing him?

10. J.T. says, "How in the world is the ice supposed to keep my hand cold with this big bandage on it?" How will the nurse reply?

11. J.T. says, "I'll be able to keep my hand up when I'm awake, but what about when I go to sleep?" What suggestion can the nurse make to help J.T. comply with the instructions?

J.T.'s recovery was uncomplicated; he received follow-up occupational therapy and regained the full use of his hand.

Case Study 13

Name ____________________ Class/Group ______ Date ______

Group Members ____________________

INSTRUCTIONS: All questions apply to this case study. Your responses should be brief and to the point. Adequate space has been provided for answers. When asked to provide several answers, they should be listed in order of priority or significance. Do not assume information that is not provided. Please print or write clearly. If your response is not legible, it will be marked as ? and you will need to rewrite it.

Scenario

Dr. C., a 53-year-old nursing professor, comes to your chronic fatigue clinic for evaluation of long-term fatigue, weakness, and pain, which have become increasingly disruptive to her lifestyle. Over the years, she sought medical advice about her fatigue but received vague and often conflicting advice such as "get more exercise," "get more rest," "eat better," "exercise more and lose weight," and "pull yourself together." Despite treatment for "depression," the fatigue remains unrelenting. Nothing seems to help. She confides in you that she is so discouraged and tired of dragging through each day that she has thought of suicide, but it violates her belief system.

1. You ask her to describe her symptoms. What questions will you ask about her fatigue, weakness, and pain?

Dr. C. describes her fatigue as daily, unrelenting, and worse in the evening. The overall fatigue, together with muscular weakness ("feels rubbery") and "nervelike" pain, is aggravated by activity and long days. She experiences nausea when extremely fatigued. She has difficulty negotiating inclines and stairs. Although rest makes her feel better, she says she feels guilty about "taking the time." She says she rarely attends social events, is having trouble doing her housekeeping, and has had to give up doing yardwork. She tells you she worries a great deal about her future and whether she'll be able to work until retirement.

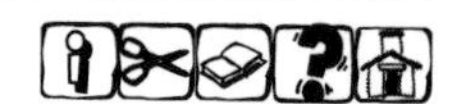

You take a detailed history in preparation for a physical and psychosocial evaluation. At age 17, she developed polio. She described this experience as sudden onset (over a 6-hour period) with fatigue, high fever (104.8° F) with shaking chills, weakness, and aching all over. The next day, she dragged her feet, experienced constipation, became anorectic, and had chills, indescribable muscle aches, and constant pain. The asymmetric muscular weakness affected all her extremities, especially her legs. This was followed by over 6 months of hospitalization featuring the Sister Kenny method of treatment. The moist, hot packs helped relieve the extreme neuromuscular pain. Together with gentle exercise (swimming pool), they helped prevent contractures. "It was that experience that motivated me to become a nurse," she said and smiled. "It has always been a point of pride that I worked so hard and overcame such a vicious disease." Based on her history and your experience with other patients, you suspect her fatigue, weakness and pain are manifestations of postpolio syndrome (PPS).

2. What comments did Dr. C. make indicating that her functional status (ability to function on a daily basis) is currently compromised? (List five.) ❍ ❍ ❍ ❍ ❍

3. What questions do you need to ask to gain an understanding of her support systems? ❍ ❍ ❍ ❍ ❍

4. Dr. C. admitted she is used to "pushing herself even when it hurts." Then she asks whether you think an exercise program would be good for her. How would you respond? ❍ ❍ ❍ ❍ ❍

5. Dr. C. undergoes some diagnostic tests to confirm the diagnosis of postpolio syndrome. What type of tests might be used for muscle evaluation?

The diagnosis of postpolio syndrome (PPS) as a source of Dr. C.'s fatigue, weakness, and pain is confirmed by the physiatrist. Dr. C. is surprised that she has never heard of PPS and that none of the other physicians have ever suggested it to her. She expresses interest in learning more about her diagnosis.

6. What resources can you suggest to her for further information?

7. On a follow-up visit, you work with Dr. C. on ways to adapt her lifestyle to her limitations. List several prosthetic devices that may help control her fatigue, weakness, and pain, and prevent further loss in muscular functioning.

8. What other suggestions can you make to help Dr. C. adapt to her limitation?

9. On her next visit, Dr. C. tells you she was "shocked" at the idea of thinking of herself as "handicapped." She adds, sadly, "I thought I had beat this years ago, but now my old enemy has come back to haunt me." How do you explain her comments?

Although this case featured someone whose poliomyelitis generally affected the lower body, others experience polio over their whole body, even affecting arm movement and breathing. Many individuals with PPS also develop trouble breathing and swallowing, so a history of polio should always be a question asked in geriatric populations and immigrants who may have been exposed to polio.

Since many health care providers today have had no experience with PPS, it is important that Dr. C. find someone who can help her identify her unique needs for anesthesia, pain management, and postoperative/preoperative care. There are some excellent Internet support resources for PPS. Some are of particularly high quality, because some health care providers had polio as children and have taken the initiative in their own self-care. Help Dr. C. identify some of these resources.

Case Study 2

Name ______________________ Class/Group ______ Date ______

Group Members ______________________________________

INSTRUCTIONS: All questions apply to this case study. Your responses should be brief and to the point. Adequate space has been provided for answers. When asked to provide several answers, they should be listed in order of priority or significance. Do not assume information that is not provided. Please print or write clearly. If your response is not legible, it will be marked as ? and you will need to rewrite it.

❍ ❍ ❍ / ❍ ❍

Scenario

T.H., a 57-year-old stockbroker, has come to the gastroenterologist for treatment of recurrent mild to severe cramping in his abdomen and blood-streaked stool. You are the RN doing his initial work-up. Your findings include a mildly obese (male-pattern obesity) man who demonstrates moderate guarding of his abdomen with both direct and rebound tenderness, especially in the LLQ. His VS are 168/98, 110, 24, 38.0° C, and he is slightly diaphoretic. T.H. reports that he has periodic constipation. He has had previous episodes of abdominal cramping, but this time the pain is getting worse. He has NKDA.

PMH: T.H. has a "sedentary job with lots of emotional moments"; he has smoked a pack of cigarettes a day for 30 years and has had "2 or 3 mixed drinks in the evening" until 2 months ago. He states, "I haven't had anything to drink in 60 days." He denies regular exercise—"Just no time." His diet consists mostly of "white bread, meat, potatoes, and ice cream with fruit and nuts over it." Denies hx of cardiac or pulmonary problems and no personal hx of cancer, although his father and older brother died of colon cancer. He takes no "regular" medications and denies the use of any other drugs.

1. Identify four general health risk problems T.H. exhibits. ❍ ❍ ❍ ❍ ❍

2. Identify a key factor in his family history that may have profound implications for his health and present state of mind? ❍ ❍ ❍ ❍ ❍

3. Identify three key findings on his physical exam, and indicate their significance. ❍ ❍ ❍ ❍ ❍

Based on physical exam and history, the physician diagnoses T.H. as having acute diverticulitis and discusses an outpatient treatment plan with him.

4. What is diverticulitis? What are the consequences of untreated diverticulitis?

5. While the patient is experiencing the severe crampy pain of acute diverticulitis, what nursing interventions would you perform to help him feel more comfortable?

6. What is the rationale for ordering bed rest?

7. What classes of medications would be prescribed for someone hospitalized for acute diverticulitis?

Metronidazole (Flagyl) or clindamycin (Cleocin) are antibiotics used in conjunction with a broad-spectrum penicillin, cephalosporin, or aminoglycoside to treat diverticulitis. T.H. is being sent home with prescriptions for Flagyl 500 mg PO q6h and amoxicillin (Augmentin) 875 mg PO bid.

8. Given his history, what questions must you ask T.H. before he takes the initial dose of Flagyl? State your rationale.

9. What is a disulfiram reaction? ❍ ❍ ❍ ❍ ❍

10. Aside from warning T.H. about the interactions just described, what instructions should you give him regarding his Flagyl prescription? ❍ ❍ ❍ ❍ ❍

11. What information would you want to know before starting T.H. on ampicillin? ❍ ❍ ❍ ❍ ❍

12. What are the s/s of an allergic reaction? ❍ ❍ ❍ ❍ ❍

13. What will you do if the patient indicates a history of an allergic reaction to PCN? ❍ ❍ ❍ ❍ ❍

14. In order to prevent future episodes of constipation, what dietary changes would the R.D. discuss with T.H.? ❍ ❍ ❍ ❍ ❍

You obtain a referral for T.H. to work with an RD about dietary issues.

15. What measures do you think the RD will discuss with T.H. to avoid recurrent acute diverticulitis?

T.H. returns for a check-up 14 days later; all s/s of diverticulitis gone. He is working on his lifestyle changes and reports he is walking 30 min qd. Only 10% to 25% of patients with diverticulitis require any surgery (usually a colectomy). Those who do often suffer recurrent uncontrollable diverticulitis.

Case Study 3

Name ______________________ Class/Group ______ Date ______

Group Members ____

INSTRUCTIONS: All questions apply to this case study. Your responses should be brief and to the point. Adequate space has been provided for answers. When asked to provide several answers, they should be listed in order of priority or significance. Do not assume information that is not provided. Please print or write clearly. If your response is not legible, it will be marked as ? and you will need to rewrite it.

Scenario

A healthy 14-year-old boy, R.K., is admitted to an outpatient clinic. About 4 hours ago, he was rollerblading and fell while jumping over some obstacles. His left arm was caught under him as he fell. He had some "sharp" pain in the LUQ immediately after the fall. This pain eased off gradually but is coming back now. His mother brought him to the clinic because he fainted every time he tried to stand up. He c/o nausea and has vomited twice. R.K. appears somewhat pale and slightly diaphoretic. He denies being SOB or dizzy when lying down. VS are 104/52 (supine), 92, 24, afebrile.

1. What are R.K.'s key symptoms?

2. What organs lie in the LUQ (left upper quadrant)?

3. What are the nurse's assessment priorities? (list in order of priority).

4. The clinic is not equipped to care for R.K. What should they do next?

5. While the nurses are waiting for the transport unit, what interventions would they initiate?

6. R.K. is sent by ambulance to your ED, which is 5 miles away. You are the RN receiving R.K. What do you do first?

7. R.K. does not have SOB, dizziness, or N/V while lying down. Given the circumstances of the accident, what is the significance of this statement?

8. R.K.'s CT scan reveals a ruptured spleen; he needs immediate surgery. What additional information do you need to obtain before he goes to the OR?

9. What is the greatest danger of a splenic rupture?

10. Before surgery, which labs should be drawn?

R.K. is taken to OR and undergoes an exploratory laparotomy and splenorrhaphy. Estimated blood loss (EBL) is 1600 ml, most of which was infused by means of the Cell Saver.

11. What is a splenorrhaphy, and why should this be done instead of a splenectomy?

12. R.K. is 14 years old, and he heals rapidly. He is discharged on the fifth postop day after having his sutures removed. What factors may have favored his wound healing?

Case Study 5

Name ______________________ Class/Group ______ Date ______

Group Members ____

INSTRUCTIONS: All questions apply to this case study. Your responses should be brief and to the point. Adequate space has been provided for answers. When asked to provide several answers, they should be listed in order of priority or significance. Do not assume information that is not provided. Please print or write clearly. If your response is not legible, it will be marked as ? and you will need to rewrite it.

Scenario

W.T., a 22-year-old white male, presented to the ED with a c/o "bad" abdominal pain. The generalized abdominal pain started 24 hours ago but seemed to "ease up" after he vomited. Several hours later the pain returned but had shifted to the RLQ and has remained there. The pain is steadily getting worse. W.T. reports marked nausea and "dry heaves," and he has no appetite. He has also had diarrhea for the last day. VS are 124/76, 92, 16, 38.8° C. W.T. works in a bar, has no health insurance, and his history is positive for tobacco ("1½ packs a day"), ETOH ("6-pack of beer a day"), and marijuana ("couple of hits a day"). He is allergic to PCN ("It makes me itch all over").

1. What organs are located in the RLQ?

2. In what order will the ED nurse examine this patient's abdomen?

3. Next, the patient's abdomen is checked for rebound tenderness. How is this done, and what does it indicate?

You note no masses and localized rebound tenderness in the RLQ. W.T.'s lab work returns: WBC 15.5 cmm with a left shift, Hgb 14.6 g/dL, Hct 43.8%, platelets 280 thou/cmm; the UA is unremarkable.

4. One of these labs is markedly abnormal and, when combined with the physical findings, is usually indicative of a specific diagnosis. Identify the abnormal lab value, the assessment findings, and probable diagnosis.

W.T. is sent to the OR for an open exploratory laparotomy for probable acute appendicitis. He undergoes an appendectomy for a purulent but unruptured appendix and is admitted to your unit at 2330. His VS are stable and his orders include: D_5½NS with 20 mEq KCl/L at 100 ml/h; cefoxitin (Mefoxin) 2 g IV q8h x 2 doses; diet as tolerated; up ad lib; morphine sulfate 5 mg prn for pain q4–6h; when tolerating PO fluid, change pain medication to Tylenol #3 1–2 PO q4h prn for pain; droperidol (Inapsine) ¼ to ½ ml IV/IM q6h prn.

5. Which of the above orders need to be clarified before a dose is given? Explain.

6. Just how will you determine the seriousness of W.T.'s allergic reaction to PCN?

7. What type of reaction is considered an allergic reaction?

8. During the morning report, you are told that W.T. has had an uneventful night; his VS are stable, and his IV of D_5½NS at 100 ml/h is infusing on time. He received his second and final dose of prophylactic cefoxitin, and he had no signs of allergic reaction. He will probably be discharged this AM. What questions do you want to ask the night nurse before she leaves?

9. Indeed, W.T. appears stable, and discharge orders are written the afternoon after surgery. What key issues need to be addressed in his discharge teaching?

Many inherent individual factors will affect the scope and direction of patient teaching. Consider W.T.'s background: he works in a bar, and his history is positive for tobacco, ETOH, and marijuana. These factors should not be glossed over. To address them would ensure the best chance of a full recovery.

10. Outline patient teaching on pain that would address these issues.

11. There are several additional areas for teaching that are not addressed in the previous questions. Can you think what they might be?

Case Study 6

Name ______________________ Class/Group ______ Date ______

Group Members ____

INSTRUCTIONS: All questions apply to this case study. Your responses should be brief and to the point. Adequate space has been provided for answers. When asked to provide several answers, they should be listed in order of priority or significance. Do not assume information that is not provided. Please print or write clearly. If your response is not legible, it will be marked as ? and you will need to rewrite it.

Scenario

While you are working as a nurse on a GI/GU floor, you receive a call from your affiliate outpatient clinic notifying you of a direct admission, ETA (estimated time of arrival) 60 minutes. She gives you the following information: A.G. is an 87-year-old woman with a 3-day history of intermittent abdominal pain, abdominal bloating, and N/V. A.G. moved from Italy to join her grandson and his family only 2 months ago and she speaks very little English. All information was obtained through her grandson. PMH: colectomy for colon cancer 6 years ago, ventral hernia repair 2 years ago. No hx of CAD, DM, or pulmonary disease. She takes only ibuprofen occasionally for mild arthritis. Allergies include sulfa drugs and meperidine. A.G.'s tentative diagnosis is small bowel obstruction (SBO) secondary to adhesions. A.G. is being admitted to your floor for diagnostic work-up. Her VS are stable, she has an IV of $D_5\frac{1}{2}NS$ with 20 mEq KCl at 100 ml/h, and 3 L O_2/nc.

1. Based on the nurse's report, what signs of bowel obstruction did A.G. present?

2. Are there other s/s that you should observe for while A.G. is in your care?

3. A.G. and her grandson arrive on your unit. You admit A.G. to her room and introduce yourself as her nurse. As her grandson interprets for her, she pats your hand. You know that you need to complete a physical examination and take a history. What will you do first?

4. The grandson, an attorney, tells you elderly Italian women are extremely modest and may not answer questions completely. How might you gather information in this case?

5. What key questions must you ask this patient while you have the use of an interpreter?

6. How would the description of A.G.'s pain differ if she has a small vs. large bowel obstruction?

7. With some difficulty, you insert an NGT into A.G. and connect it to intermittent LWS. How will you check for placement of the NGT? ❍ ❍ ❍ ❍ ❍

8. List, in order, the structures through which the NGT must pass as it is inserted. ❍ ❍ ❍ ❍ ❍

9. What comfort measures are important for A.G. while she has an NGT? ❍ ❍ ❍ ❍ ❍

10. You note that A.G.'s NGT has not drained in the last 3 hours. What can you do to facilitate drainage? ❍ ❍ ❍ ❍ ❍

11. The NGT suddenly drains 575 ml; then it slows down to about 250 ml/2h. Is this an expected amount?

12. You enter A.G.'s room to initiate your shift assessment. A.G. has been hospitalized 3 days and her abdomen seems to be more distended than yesterday. How would you determine whether A.G.'s abdominal distention has changed?

After 3 days of NGT suction, A.G.'s symptoms are unrelieved. She reports continued nausea, crampy, and sometimes very strong abdominal pain; her hand grips are weaker; and she seems to be increasingly lethargic. You look up her latest laboratory values and compare them with the admission data. Her Na has changed from 136 to 130 mmol/L, K has changed from 3.7 to 2.5 mmol/L, Cl from 108 to 97 mmol/L, CO_2 25 to 31 mmol/L, BUN from 19 to 38 mg/dL, creatinine from 1 to 2.2 mg/dL, glucose 126 to 65 mg/dL, albumin from 3.0 to 2.1 g/dL, and protein from 6.8 to 4.9 g/dL.

13. Which lab values are of concern to you? Why?

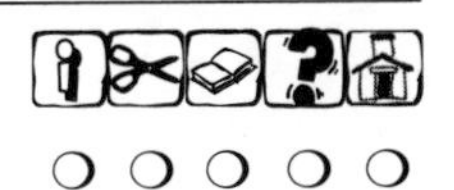

14. What measures do you anticipate to correct each of the imbalances described in question #13?

In view of A.G.'s continued slow deterioration, the surgeon meets with the patient and her family and they agree to surgery. The surgeon releases an 18-inch section of proximal ileum that has been constricted by adhesions. Several areas looked ischemic, so these were excised, and an end-to-end anastomosis was done. A.G. tolerated the procedure well and recovered rapidly from the anesthesia in the postanesthesia care unit (PACU). Once on the unit, her recovery was slow but steady. A.G. went home in the care of her grandson and his wife on the seventh postop day. Discharge plans included walking several times per day in the house; importance of cough and deep breathing (C&DB) and use of the incentive spirometer (IS) q2h; and observing the wound for s/s of infection.

In reviewing the beginning of this case, it is clear that A.G.'s nutritional status has been poor. It would be appropriate for her to have a medical nutrition therapy regarding long-term nutrient needs. Be sure the grandson is included in any plans.

Case Study 7

Name ____________________ Class/Group ______ Date ______

Group Members ____________________________________

INSTRUCTIONS: All questions apply to this case study. Your responses should be brief and to the point. Adequate space has been provided for answers. When asked to provide several answers, they should be listed in order of priority or significance. Do not assume information that is not provided. Please print or write clearly. If your response is not legible, it will be marked as ? and you will need to rewrite it.

❍ ❍ ❍ / ❍ ❍

Scenario

P.M., a 24-year-old house painter, has been too ill to work for the last 3 days. When he arrives at your outpatient clinic, he seems an alert but acutely ill young man of average build, with a deep tan over exposed areas of skin. He reports headaches, severe myalgia, a low-grade fever, cough, anorexia, and N/V, especially after eating any fatty food. P.M. describes vague abdominal pain that started about the same time as the other problems. PMH: no health problems, nonsmoker, drinks a "few" beers each evening to relax. Assessment: VS are 128/84, 88, 26, 38.1° C; AAO x 3, MAEW except for aching pain in his muscles; very slight scleral jaundice present; heart tones clear and without adventitious sounds; breath sounds clear throughout A&P; abdomen soft and palpable without distinct masses. You note moderate hepatomegaly; liver edge is easily palpated and tender to palpation. P.M. mentions that his urine has been getting darker over the last 2 days.

P.M. is presenting with the key signs of hepatitis. Lab work is sent for identification of his precise problem. Results: Na 140 mmol/L, K 3.9 mmol/L, Cl 102 mmol/L, CO_2 26 mmol/L, BUN 10 mg/dL, creatinine 1.0 mg/dL, platelets 86 cmm, direct bilirubin 1.6 mg/dL, total bilirubin 2.3 mg/dL, albumin 3.8 g/dL, total protein 6.2 g/dL, ALT (SGPT) 66 U/L, AST (SGOT) 52 U/L, LDH 205 U/L, ALP 176 U/L, PT = 12 s/INR = 1.06, PTT 32 s, urine urobilinogen 1.6 E U/L, albuminuria 160 mg/dl, + bilirubinuria, + for anti-HAV IgM.

1. Which key diagnostic tests will determine exactly what type of hepatitis is present? ❍ ❍ ❍ ❍ ❍

2. An acute care battery was drawn. Which of the labs listed above specifically indicates liver disease? ❍ ❍ ❍ ❍ ❍

3. List eight or more drugs that can cause increased ALT levels.

4. Considering that the basic pathology of hepatitis involves inflammation, degeneration, and regeneration of the hepatocyte, what type of diet will you strongly encourage P.M. to follow?

5. Differentiate between hepatitis A, B, and C on the basis of the mode of transmission and prevention.

6. Name three major activities that can be done in a community to prevent the spread of hepatitis (any/all types).

7. In P.M.'s case, the IgM-class anti-HAV antibody is positive. This indicates that P.M. is infected with hepatitis A and is in the acute or early convalescent period of the disease. Is this disease contagious? What precaution would you take?

8. Pruritus is usually associated with jaundice. What will you do to ease this problem for P.M.?

9. How would you explain to P.M. the likely progression of his disease? (requires not only knowledge of disease and progression but figuring out his thought processes)

10. P.M. is living at home with his parents and 8 younger siblings. The youngest is a 4-year-old. His parents ask how to prevent the rest of the family from getting hepatitis. What specific instructions will you give? How will you know that these instructions are understood?

11. Given P.M.'s lifestyle, what specific patient teaching points must you emphasize?

12. List four critical issues relevant to P.M.'s nursing care.

Case Study 8

Name ______________________ Class/Group ______ Date ______

Group Members ________________________________

INSTRUCTIONS: All questions apply to this case study. Your responses should be brief and to the point. Adequate space has been provided for answers. When asked to provide several answers, they should be listed in order of priority or significance. Do not assume information that is not provided. Please print or write clearly. If your response is not legible, it will be marked as ? and you will need to rewrite it.

Scenario

John Doe #6, an approximately 50-year-old man, is admitted to your floor from the ED. He is lethargic, has a cachectic appearance, does not follow commands consistently, and is mildly combative when aroused. He smells strongly of alcohol and has a notably swollen abdomen and lower extremities. This man was sent to the ED by local police who found him lying unresponsive along a rural road. He was aroused somewhat in the ED. Examination and x-rays are negative for any injury, and he is admitted to your unit for observation. He has no ID and is not awake enough to give any history or to coherently answer questions. Admitting orders are: admit to E3 with R/O hepatic encephalopathy; IV D_5½NS with 20 mEq KCl at 75 ml/h; add 1 amp MVI (multivitamins) to each L IVF (IV fluid); Foley catheter to DD (down drain); HOB at 30 to 45 degrees at all times; tap water enemas until clear; abdominal ultrasound in AM; hemogram with diff, acute care battery, NH3 now and in AM; soft restraints prn; vitamin K 10 mg IV or PO qd x 3 doses; thiamine 1 g IM qd; folic acid 5 mg IM qd; pyridoxine 100 mg PO qd; low-protein diet, eat with assistance only; call HO for any sign GI bleed, DTs, or SBP >140 or <100, DBP <50, P >120.

1. Which of the above orders must be done by the RN? By the aide? By the clerk?

2. The lab work drawn in the ED has come back. The blood alcohol level (BAL) is 320 mg/dL, and the blood ammonia (NH_3) level is 85 μg/dL. What do these values indicate?

While you are getting John Doe #6 settled, you continue your assessment. Neuro: PERRL, MAE sluggishly, pulling away during assessment, follows commands sporadically. CV: P regular but tachy without adventitious sounds. All peripheral pulses palpable and 3+ bilat, 3+ pitting edema in lower extremities. IV of D_5½NS with 20 mEq KCl/L at 75 ml/h in L forearm. Resp: breath sounds decreased to all lobes, no adventitious sounds audible, patient does not cooperate with C&DB, on RA (room air) with SaO_2 at 90%. GI: tongue and gums are beefy red and swollen, abdomen enlarged and protuberant, girth is 141 cm (64 in), abdominal skin is taut and slightly tender to palpation. BS x 4 quads. GU: Foley to DD with 75 ml dark amber urine since admission (2 h). Skin: color pale to torso and LEs (lower extremities), heavily sunburned to UEs (upper extremities) and head. Skin appears thin and dry. Numerous spider angiomas on upper abdomen with several dilated veins across abdomen. VS are 120/60, 104, 32, 37.3° C. His protein is 5.2 g/dL, and albumin is 2.9 g/dL. A toxicology screen and electrolytes have been drawn.

3. What is the significance of the spider angiomas, dilated abdominal veins, peripheral edema, and distended abdomen?

4. How would you further assess the distended abdomen, and what is the clinical name for your findings?

5. What is your concern about John Doe's nutritional status? What are your objective reasons?

6. Why is the low-protein diet ordered? How much protein is reasonable?

7. How might you respond to fellow staff nurses' remarks, "Why are we wasting time with this 'wino?' He isn't worth the time or money. Why don't they let him die?"

8. A nursing problem relative to John Doe's care is "risk for injury." Ensuring safety is a critical part of the nursing role. Consider at least three areas of injury risk, and identify actions you will take to ensure his safety.

9. What are the s/s of delirium tremens (DTs)?

10. Falls are particularly dangerous for someone in this patient's situation. Why?

11. The aide asks you why the patient has tap water enemas ordered and how many to do "until clear." How would you reply?

John Doe #6 survives a rocky course of hepatic encephalopathy and near-renal failure. After 27 days, including a week in the ICU, he is discharged to a drug and alcohol rehabilitation facility. He is employed as a longshoreman; fortunately, his insurance covers his month of in-house intense rehabilitation.

Case Study 9

Name ______________________ Class/Group ______ Date ______

Group Members ______________________________________

INSTRUCTIONS: All questions apply to this case study. Your responses should be brief and to the point. Adequate space has been provided for answers. When asked to provide several answers, they should be listed in order of priority or significance. Do not assume information that is not provided. Please print or write clearly. If your response is not legible, it will be marked as ? and you will need to rewrite it.

Scenario

J.S., a 57-year-old salesman, has come to his practitioner's office with a moderate amount of chest pain. He says this pain comes and goes and is worst at night, when it wakes him up. He looks haggard, with dark circles under his eyes, "I've got to get more sleep than this."

1. What are some common causes of "chest pain?"

2. What will you ask J.S. to better evaluate his pain?

3. J.S. says the pain has been waking him up for 3 months. What would you want to know about J.S.'s lifestyle?

J.S. indicates that he has tried taking antacids and some other medicine he bought at the drug store just in case these were ulcers, but he gets no relief. He tried some sleeping pills, but he just woke up groggy with a headache in addition to the chest pain.

4. What tests will be done to help determine the source of the problem?

5. A barium swallow confirms a large sliding esophageal hiatal hernia. J.S. asks, "What is a hiatal hernia, and what do you mean it's sliding?" How would you explain this to him?

6. J.S. asks, "Is 'heartburn' always caused by a hiatal hernia?" How would you respond?

7. J.S. would rather try more conservative medical treatment before having surgery. What measures can he try to minimize his pain? List at least five.

J.S. writes down all your instructions and is determined to conquer his problem without surgery.

8. What meds are most likely to be prescribed for J.S.? What will he need to know about them? ❍ ❍ ❍ ❍ ❍

Two months later J.S. reappears at your office, looking even worse than before. "I just can't keep the pain controlled, especially when I'm on the road."

9. After discussion, J.S. agrees on a date to have his hiatal hernia repaired. As he does this, he looks doubtful but desperate. What do you want to ask him right now? ❍ ❍ ❍ ❍ ❍

10. J.S. wants to know how the minilaparotomy (minilap) surgery is different from the larger laparotomy surgery. Using a picture you explain the following: ❍ ❍ ❍ ❍ ❍

11. J.S. is to have a minilap. What preop teaching will he need? ❍ ❍ ❍ ❍ ❍

J.S. went to surgery for an NFP by means of a minilap. The surgery was successful, and J.S. went home on the second day postop. Two months later he stops back in when he comes in for an appointment with his surgeon. He has had complete relief of his gastric reflux and can sleep flat at night without waking up.

Case Study 10

Name ______________________ Class/Group ______ Date ______

Group Members ______________________________________

INSTRUCTIONS: All questions apply to this case study. Your responses should be brief and to the point. Adequate space has been provided for answers. When asked to provide several answers, they should be listed in order of priority or significance. Do not assume information that is not provided. Please print or write clearly. If your response is not legible, it will be marked as ? and you will need to rewrite it.

❍ ❍ ❍ / ❍ ❍

Scenario

J.D., with 2 years of sobriety behind him, has been promoted from longshoreman to nightshift foreman in a warehouse. He has new hope and new friends in his AA groups. Unfortunately, his cirrhotic liver has not recovered from 20 years of heavy drinking, and he still has residual effects. During the past 2 days he has had a "bad cough." This morning he coughed up bright red blood (BRB) and came into the ED. His coughing and bleeding have subsided for now. An IV of $D_5\frac{1}{2}$NS with 20 KCl/L at 100 ml/h is started and baseline labs are drawn. He is sent to the floor for observation. Shortly after you admit J.D., you hear coughing while passing his room. You enter and see BRB all over his gown and bed. He looks very frightened.

1. What needs to be done at once? ❍ ❍ ❍ ❍ ❍

2. What specific tasks must be done? ❍ ❍ ❍ ❍ ❍

3. What do you think J.D.'s emotional state is? How would his body respond to this emotion? ❍ ❍ ❍ ❍ ❍

4. Recognizing his emotional state, what can you do to intervene? ❍ ❍ ❍ ❍ ❍

5. What treatment options exist for esophageal varices? List in the order in which they are most likely to be tried. ❍ ❍ ❍ ❍ ❍

6. The gastroenterologist comes to the unit to perform an endoscopic exam. How will you prepare J.D. for this? ❍ ❍ ❍ ❍ ❍

7. The gastroenterologist performs the fiberoptic endoscopic examination. Neither cauterization nor sclerotherapy is successful for more than a few minutes and J.D.'s bleeding intensifies. The physician elects to use balloon tamponade to hold pressure on the varices until J.D. can more safely undergo surgery. What key rule will you observe with this tube? ❍ ❍ ❍ ❍ ❍

8. What is the major complication of balloon tamponade, and how can you help prevent this? ❍ ❍ ❍ ❍ ❍

9. J.D. looks at you and asks, “Am I going to die?” You know that the operative mortality is 5% to 15% in elective cases and 50% in emergency cases. Even the survivors have a curtailed lifespan because of an increased rate of hepatic encephalopathy and liver failure. How would you respond?

10. What is shunt surgery and why is it done?

11. J.D.'s current H/H = 8.6/26. He is to receive 2 units of PRCs and 2 units of albumin (SPA). How will you know if J.D. is having any negative reactions to the transfusion, and what would you do to intervene?

12. How much will you expect the hematocrit to rise after the transfusion of 2 units of PRCs?

The blood has infused without evidence of reaction, and his VS are stable. J.D. talked to the hospital chaplain at length and then was sent to OR for a portocaval shunt. He will be transferred to ICU afterward for recovery.

Case Study 11

Name ________________________ Class/Group ______ Date ______

Group Members ____

INSTRUCTIONS: All questions apply to this case study. Your responses should be brief and to the point. Adequate space has been provided for answers. When asked to provide several answers, they should be listed in order of priority or significance. Do not assume information that is not provided. Please print or write clearly. If your response is not legible, it will be marked as ? and you will need to rewrite it.

Scenario

C.W., a 36-year-old woman, was admitted several days ago with a diagnosis of recurrent inflammatory bowel disease (IBD) and possible small bowel obstruction (SBO). C.W. is married, and her husband and 11-year-old son are very supportive, but she has no extended family in-state. She has IBD x 15 years and has been on prednisone 40 mg qd for the last 5 years. She is very thin; at 5'2" she weighs 86 lb and has lost 40 lb over the last 10 years. She has an average of 5 to 10 loose stools per day. C.W.'s life has gradually become dominated by her disease (anorexia; lactase deficiency; profound fatigue; frequent nausea and diarrhea; frequent hospitalizations for dehydration; and recurring, crippling abdominal pain that often strikes unexpectedly). The pain is incapacitating and relieved only by a small dose of diazepam (Valium), Pedialyte, and total bed rest. She confides in you that sexual activity is difficult, "It always causes diarrhea, nausea, and lots of pain. It's difficult for both of us." She is so weak she cannot stand without help. You write CBR (complete bed rest) with side rails up on the Kardex. (You also make a mental note of the probability that she has osteoporosis secondary to long-term steroid use.

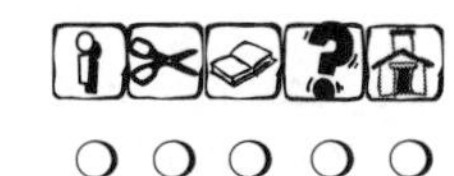

1. Identify six priority problems for C.W.

2. You enter C.W.'s room and note that she has been crying. You ask what's wrong, and she explains that the nurse who admitted her to the hospital the last time said, "Welcome to death row!" C.W. says that she is knowledgeable about her condition, but she still can't seem to shake that "death row" feeling. She was afraid to come to the hospital this time. What can you do to help this woman?

C.W. replies, "Treat me with respect, and as a person, not a disease. Act like I have the right and intelligence to understand my condition. Recognize that I probably know what I'm talking about when I try to refuse a delicious milkshake. When I'm either NPO or nauseated, please don't pop popcorn where I can smell it! It's pure torture!"

3. Considering C.W.'s weakness, chronic diarrhea, and lower-than-desired body weight, what interventions should minimize skin breakdown?

C.W.'s condition deteriorates on the third day postadmission; she experiences intractable abdominal pain and unrelenting N/V. C.W. is taken to the OR for probable SBO and is readmitted to your unit from the postanesthesia care unit (PACU). 38 inches of her small bowel were found to be severely stenosed with 2 areas of visible perforation. Much of the remaining bowel is severely inflamed and friable. A total of 5 feet of distal ileum and 2 feet of colon have been removed and a temporary ileostomy established. She has a Jackson-Pratt (JP) drain to bulb suction in her RLQ and her wound was packed and left open. She has 2 peripheral IVs, an NGT, and a Foley. Her VS are 112/72, 86, 24, 38.2° C (tympanic).

4. You review the postop orders before the physician leaves the unit. One order reads vitamin A at 25,000 IU/d x 10 days. Why is C.W. to receive vitamin A?

5. You begin a thorough postop assessment of C.W.'s abdomen. What does your assessment include? List these in the order in which the assessment should be completed.

6. A nursing student enters C.W.'s room and auscultates her abdomen. She looks at you and excitedly announces that she hears good bowel sounds. You take the opportunity to teach her the proper method of auscultating bowel sounds on a patient who has NGT to continuous LWS. How would you correct her error?

The nursing student follows your advice and listens again. She says "You're right, I didn't hear a thing." You tell her that she can impress her classmates while educating them in the correct technique.

7. C.W. is 4 days postop. During the routine dressing change, you note a small pool of yellow green drainage in the deepest part of the wound. You realize the physician will want a wound culture. How will you culture C.W.'s wound?

8. You obtain a wound culture, complete the dressing change, obtain a full set of VS and note a temp of 38.1° C, and assess increased tenderness in C.W.'s abdomen. You call to notify the physician and ask for additional orders. What orders do you anticipate?

9. What information do you need to send to the lab with the wound culture specimen?

10. The physician calls back and asks you to describe C.W.'s wound. What key aspects of the wound should be included?

11. The physician asks you how C.W.'s stoma and drainage look. What should a healthy stoma and usual drainage look like?

12. Will any aspect of C.W.'s history significantly affect the wound healing process? How?

13. With a fairly significant wound infection developing, why is C.W.'s temperature relatively low?

14. The physician tells you that she will be over to examine C.W. As you tell C.W. that her doctor is coming to talk to her, C.W. says that she feels something wet running down her side. You find the some leakage of intestinal drainage onto the skin. What should you do?

You change the ileostomy appliance before the physician arrives. C.W. is evaluated, and it is determined that she should return to surgery for exploratory laparotomy.

Case Study 12

Name ______________________ Class/Group ______ Date ______

Group Members ______________________________________

INSTRUCTIONS: All questions apply to this case study. Your responses should be brief and to the point. Adequate space has been provided for answers. When asked to provide several answers, they should be listed in order of priority or significance. Do not assume information that is not provided. Please print or write clearly. If your response is not legible, it will be marked as ? and you will need to rewrite it.

Scenario (Continuation of Case 11)

C.W. is a 36-year-old woman admitted 7 days ago for IBD with SBO. She underwent surgery 3 days postadmission for a colectomy and ileostomy. She developed peritonitis and 4 days later returned to the OR for an exploratory laparotomy. The lap revealed another area of perforated bowel, generalized peritonitis, and a fistula tract to the abdominal surface. Another 12 inches of ileum were resected (total of 7 feet of ileum and 2 feet of colon). The peritoneal cavity was irrigated with NS, and 3 tubes were placed: a JP drain to bulb suction, a rubber catheter to irrigate the wound bed with NS, and a sump drain to remove the irrigation. The initial JP drain remains in place. A R subclavian triple lumen catheter was inserted.

1. C.W. returns from PACU on your shift. What do you do when her bed is rolled into her room?

2. You pull the covers back to inspect the abdominal dressing and find that the original surgical dressing is saturated with fresh bloody drainage. What should you do?

3. C.W. has a total of 4 tubes in her abdomen as well as an NGT. What information do you want to know about each tube?

Note: For safety, all tubes should be clearly labeled.

4. The sump irrigation fluid bag is nearly empty. You close the roller clamp, thread the IV tubing through the infusion pump, check the irrigation catheter connection site to make sure it is snug, and then discover that the nearly empty liter bag infusing into C.W.'s abdomen is D_5W, not NS. Does this require any action? If so, give rationale for actions, and explain the overall situation.

The physician arrives on the unit and removes C.W.'s surgical dressing. There is a small "bleeder" at the edge of the incision, so the physician calls for a suture and ties off the bleeder. You take the opportunity to ask her about a morphine PCA pump for C.W., and the physician says she will go write the orders right away.

5. Postop pain will be a problem for C.W. after the anesthesia wears off. How do you plan to address this?

6. Pharmacy delivers C.W.'s first bag of TPN. The physician has written for you to start the TPN at a rate of 60 ml/h and decrease the maintenance IV rate by the same amount. What is the purpose of this order?

7. The physician did not specifically order glucose monitoring, but you know that it should be initiated. You plan to conduct a finger stick q2h for the first several hours. What is your rationale?

8. C.W.'s blood glucose increased temporarily, but by the next day it dropped to an average of 70 to 80 mg/dL and has remained there for 2 days. Her VS are stable, but her abdominal wound shows no signs of healing. She has lost 1 kg over the 3 days. What do these data mean?

You discuss your concerns with C.W.'s physician, and she agrees to request a consult from an RD. After gathering data and making several calculations, the RD makes recommendations to the attending physician. The TPN orders are adjusted, C.W. begins to gain weight slowly, and her wound shows signs of healing. Nutritional problems in clinical populations can be complex and often require special attention.

9. You and a coworker read the following in C.W.'s progress notes: "Wound healing by secondary closure. Formation of granular tissue with epithelialization noted around edges. Have requested dietitian to consult on ongoing basis. Will continue to follow." Your coworker turns to you and asks whether you know what that means. How would you explain?

10. Both of you start to discuss what specific digestive difficulties C.W. is likely to face in the future. What problems might C.W. be prone to develop after having so much of her bowel removed?

11. The RD consults with C.W. about dietary needs. You attend the session so that you will be able to reinforce the information. What basic information is the dietitian likely to discuss with C.W.?

12. After 3 days of dressing changes, C.W.'s skin is quite irritated, and a small skin tear has appeared where tape was removed. How can you minimize this type of skin breakdown and help this area heal?

13. What specifics of ostomy teaching do you plan to do.

C.W. successfully battled peritonitis. Gradually, tubes were removed as she grew stronger with TPN and time. C.W. learned how to change her ostomy appliance and was discharged to home.

Case Study 13

Name ______________________ Class/Group ______ Date ______

Group Members ______________________________________

INSTRUCTIONS: All questions apply to this case study. Your responses should be brief and to the point. Adequate space has been provided for answers. When asked to provide several answers, they should be listed in order of priority or significance. Do not assume information that is not provided. Please print or write clearly. If your response is not legible, it will be marked as ? and you will need to rewrite it.

❍ ❍ ❍ / ❍ ❍

Scenario

B.B., a 72-year-old woman, is admitted from the ED with c/o constant, severe abdominal and lower back pain x 2 days and SOB over the last 24 hours. "I've had to rest 4 or 5 times gettin' back to the house from the shed. It's gotten real hard to manage all by myself." A niece stopped by and insisted B.B. come into the county hospital ED. B.B. has never received any medical care of any kind. She lives by herself "up the mountain" off of a dirt road in rural Pennsylvania. She is restless, nauseated, and in pain. Everything around her in the hospital is new and frightening to her. VS are 108/72, 128, 30, 37.9° C (tympanic), SaO_2 84% on 2 L O_2/nc. B.B. is admitted to your unit at 1900.

1. What possible diagnoses would you suspect with a presentation of severe abdominal pain? ❍ ❍ ❍ ❍ ❍

2. The ED nurse giving you report says that B.B.'s admitting diagnosis is R/O pancreatitis. You know that pain control is difficult in patients with pancreatitis. What information will you want to ask the ED nurse before hanging up? ❍ ❍ ❍ ❍ ❍

3. B.B. arrives on your unit. As she is getting into bed, you notice that her eyes are very wide and she is looking all around. She seems totally overwhelmed in response to the ED nurse's instructions about how to operate the bed. What of the above information may be used to guide the manner in which you approach B.B.? ❍ ❍ ❍ ❍ ❍

4. What approach would you use to obtain a psychosocial history and complete your assessment?

You complete an assessment and note the following abnormalities: restless, prefers to sit on side of bed, leaning forward and tightly clutching her handbag. States pain has decreased "some after that lady jabbed me with that needle downstairs." Skin cool, diaphoretic, and pale. Heart rate irregular and tachy. Peripheral pulses weakly palpable x 4 extremities. Resp rapid but unlabored on 2 L O_2/nc, SaO_2 85%, breath sounds absent at the base of the LLL (left lower lobe) posteriorly. Reports marked nausea without emesis. BS hypoactive x 4 quads. Abdomen distended and exquisitely tender throughout to light palpation, guarding noted. Has not voided but states that she has "made less water than usual." Poor skin turgor, dry mucous membranes, mild scleral jaundice.

5. How are you going to assess B.B.'s pain?

B.B.'s admission labs return: Na 148 mmol/L, WBC 17.2 thou/cmm, amylase 200 U/L, K 4.2 mmol/L, Hgb 12.5 g/dL, Hct 38%, lipase 375 U/L, Cl 114 mmol/L, LDH 160 U/L, HCO_3 98 mmol/L, platelets 306 cmm, AST 54 U/L, BUN 26 mg/d,; ALT 46 U/L, creatinine 1.0 mg/dL, ALP 96 U/L, glucose 185 mg/dL. You make a mental notice that calcium is missing from the list and an order for a calcium level should be obtained.

6. Indicate which lab values are important in the diagnosis of pancreatitis. ❍ ❍ ❍ ❍ ❍

7. Review the hemogram and BMP results. What results are consistent with your observations on her physical exam? ❍ ❍ ❍ ❍ ❍

8. B.B. voids 150 ml dark brown urine 2 hours after admission to your unit. What will you do? ❍ ❍ ❍ ❍ ❍

9. The physician orders a 500-ml bolus of NS and Foley to down drain. What do these orders mean, and why are they appropriate at this time? What priority assessment must be done when a fluid bolus is given? ❍ ❍ ❍ ❍ ❍

You deliver the NS bolus over an hour and insert a Foley catheter. You are surprised that the color of B.B.'s urine is dark amber, instead of the dark brown urine that you saw in the commode. You send a specimen to the lab.

10. The next time you answer B.B.'s call light, she states that her pain is, "Getting bad again." You are puzzled because she is not used to taking narcotics and it has been only 2 hours since her last injection of morphine 5 mg. What can be done to improve her pain management? ❍ ❍ ❍ ❍ ❍

NSAIDs are added to the pain regimen. You administer the first dose and notice that her bedpan is under the covers and it contains the same dark brown fluid that you noted in the commode. You ask B.B. about it and she states, "Aw honey, that's just my chewing tobacco." She spits, and the dark fluid lands in the pan.

11. Is there any connection between heavy tobacco use and the effectiveness of medicationsl?

12. Based on your discovery, what action would you take?

13. B.B.'s oximeter alarms at 83% saturated, her respiratory rate is 34, and the IV bolus has infused. You auscultate no breath sounds from the scapula down on the L. You percuss B.B.'s lung posteriorly and hear a dull thud up to the scapula on the L and percuss resonant on the R. What is the significance of your findings?

14. What two actions would you take next and why?

The physician orders a STAT CXR, which shows a significant pleural effusion developing over the LLL.

15. Based on the diagnosis of pleural effusion, what treatment will the physician likely perform next, and what is your responsibility throughout the treatment?

Patients with subdiaphragmatic inflammatory processes frequently present with pneumonia or pleural effusion. Cloudy, yellow fluid (250 ml) was removed. B.B. was placed on broad-spectrum antibiotics until the cultures returned. She was found to have acute pancreatitis and was eventually released to home. As she is wheeled out of the hospital, B.B. tells you, "I'll die up on my mountain before I'll come back here." She probably did.

Case Study 3

Name ______________________ Class/Group ______ Date ______

Group Members ____

INSTRUCTIONS: All questions apply to this case study. Your responses should be brief and to the point. Adequate space has been provided for answers. When asked to provide several answers, they should be listed in order of priority or significance. Do not assume information that is not provided. Please print or write clearly. If your response is not legible, it will be marked as ? and you will need to rewrite it.

❍ ❍ ❍ / ❍ ❍

Scenario

M.J., a 36-year-old white female, comes into the homeless shelter clinic where you work as an RN. She says she needs a prescription for birth control pills to help with her "cramps." She says she is from out of state, "between jobs," and tells you her boyfriend threw her out last night. She says she has 2 children who live with her mother "back home" and tells you she's had 3 "miscarriages." Her LMP was "3 to 4 months ago and irregular, but I don't think I'm pregnant." She denies any chronic conditions or current health problems. Her knowledge of family health history is sketchy. You smell cigarette smoke on her clothing, and she admits to smoking 2 packs of cigarettes a day. She vehemently denies ETOH and drug use and says she does not take any prescription or over-the-counter medication. Her hair is dull, and her skin is dry and sallow. She appears to be hyperalert and oriented x 3; her eyes dart around the room nervously. You watch her eyes as she looks around the room: the pupil sizes appear to respond appropriately to the ambient light and are equal bilaterally. She is 5'6" but weighs only 106 lb. Although it is a hot and humid day, she is wearing blue jeans and a man's long-sleeved flannel shirt. When she responds to your request to roll up her sleeve so you can take her VS, you notice she's watching your face for any sign of a reaction. Her arm is covered with bruises that range in color from yellow and yellow-green to brown and blue. As you insert the thermometer into her mouth, you make a mental note of several scars and bruises on her face and a recent cut on her lip. Her teeth do not appear to have been cared for in a long time.

1. How would you summarize the above information for the chart? ❍ ❍ ❍ ❍ ❍

2. List three reasons she may be requesting the oral contraceptives. ❍ ❍ ❍ ❍ ❍

3. From the previous description, state three pieces of information that indicate M.J. is malnourished.

In all clinical settings you encounter individuals who are fearful and suspicious of health care workers as part of "the system." Because of their past experiences, these persons are hypervigilant to the possibility or perception of harm, insult, or betrayal. This includes victims with a background of domestic or political abuse, prisoners, homeless, illegal aliens, non-U.S. citizens (particularly if police and health care workers worked together to torture or interrogate), and minority groups. Often there are questions you would like to ask patients, but it is necessary to wait until you have been able to build an atmosphere of trust.

4. List four questions you would like to ask someone like M.J., if you knew it wouldn't threaten her.

5. You are very concerned about the possibility of abuse, but you want to approach the question gently so you don't frighten M.J.. Instead of asking her directly about her bruises and scars, what other questions could you use that might be less threatening and could lead you to what you need to know?

The family nurse practitioner (FNP) comes in and introduces herself to M.J. She sits eye-to-eye and asks M.J. a few questions about how she has been feeling. She asks M.J. if she ever had a vaginal exam performed in the past and how it made her feel. She explains to M.J. that she would like to do a physical and vaginal exam as part of the evaluation. The FNP and you leave the room to give M.J. privacy for changing into the examination gown.

6. Explain why the FNP talked with M.J. first, before having her change into the examination gown. ❍ ❍ ❍ ❍ ❍

7. As you present your assessment to her, the FNP tells you that M.J. is not an appropriate candidate for OCs because of her age and her smoking. Explain the rationale behind this statement. ❍ ❍ ❍ ❍ ❍

8. The FNP tells you that her goal is to see whether M.J. will allow her to test for HIV status, pregnancy, TB, and STDs; take an H&H; and do a Pap smear. Explain the rationale for each of these tests in the current setting. ❍ ❍ ❍ ❍ ❍

As the FNP is setting up for her examination of M.J., she explains what she is going to do and how it should feel. She also explains the tests she would like to do and why they would be important to M.J. She makes it clear that there is no charge for the tests. During the course of the examination, M.J. admits that she has not eaten a good meal "for longer than she can remember." She also admits that her ex-boyfriend really was her pimp and he beat her when she didn't bring in enough money. She is afraid he is going to come after her and kill her if she tells anyone about their real relationship. She doesn't know anyone she can trust. M.J. says her mother "got custody of the kids several years ago while I was on crack and got sent-up for possession" and won't talk to her. M.J. also implies she will be engaging in further prostitution by saying, "I gotta earn a living the only way I know how." About your offer to teach her about condoms, she says, "It's OK, honey. I've heard it all."

M.J. allows the tests to be taken. The pregnancy test is negative. The FNP encourages her to come back for the test results and check-up. The FNP also gives her a pass for a good meal and directions to the domestic violence shelter for the night. As M.J. goes out the door, she turns to you both and says, "Hey, thanks. You've been real nice to me."

M.J. fails to keep her follow-up appointment the following week. Unfortunately, 10 days later, her body is found along the interstate. She had been sexually molested and bludgeoned to death. No one ever claims the body, and no one is ever arrested or charged in her death.

Case Study 4

Name ______________________ Class/Group ______ Date ______

Group Members ______________________________________

INSTRUCTIONS: All questions apply to this case study. Your responses should be brief and to the point. Adequate space has been provided for answers. When asked to provide several answers, they should be listed in order of priority or significance. Do not assume information that is not provided. Please print or write clearly. If your response is not legible, it will be marked as ? and you will need to rewrite it.

Scenario

You are working on a medical-surgical floor when you assume the care of K.S., a 52-year-old man who is 3 days postop from an appendectomy. K.S. was admitted to the hospital with acute R lower quadrant pain and R/O appendicitis. During surgery it was noted K.S.'s appendix had ruptured and he experienced a brief episode of hypotension. Hemostasis was immediately restored and he has been stable since that time. K.S.'s VS are 106/70, 88, 12, 100.8° F. His most recent laboratory data are Na 144 mmol/L, K 4.8 mmol/L, Cl 100 mmol/L, CO_2 25 mmol/L, BUN 84 mg/dL, creatinine 8.4 mg/dL, glucose 106 mg/dL. Yesterday, K.S.'s physician recorded in his progress note that K.S. had acute tubular necrosis (ATN).

1. What is ATN?

2. What are the implications of K.S.'s diagnosis on medications?

K.S.'s medications include gentamicin (Garamycin) 60 mg IVPB q48h. MSO_4 1–3 mg IV q4h prn for pain, and acetaminophen (Tylenol) 650 mg q4h prn for fever.

3. K.S. has three potential causes for ATN. What are they?

4. K.S. informs you he is having incisional pain. What information should you assess before administering the MSO_4 that is ordered?

5. What correlation do rising creatinine levels have with the number of functioning nephrons?

6. K.S.'s BUN and creatinine are markedly elevated. Do these elevations correlate with his risk for developing chronic renal failure?

7. S.M. calls you into his room and states, "My arm hurts where the IV is." What should you do?

8. You inspect S.M.'s IV site and note the site has no erythema, drainage, or swelling. The IV infuses freely when the dial a flow is wide open. S.M. continues to c/o tenderness at the site. What is another potential cause for his pain, and what are appropriate nursing interventions?

9. What are general nursing priorities for patients in ATN?

Case Study 5

Name ______________________ Class/Group ______ Date ______

Group Members ______________________________________

INSTRUCTIONS: All questions apply to this case study. Your responses should be brief and to the point. Adequate space has been provided for answers. When asked to provide several answers, they should be listed in order of priority or significance. Do not assume information that is not provided. Please print or write clearly. If your response is not legible, it will be marked as ? and you will need to rewrite it.

❍ ❍ ❍ / ❍ ❍

Scenario

You are working in the ED when M.B., a 72-year-old man, enters with a CC of inability to void. His initial VS are 168/92, 70, 20.

1. Are M.B.'s VS appropriate for a man his age? If not, what are the abnormalities and offer possibilities for the abnormality. ❍ ❍ ❍ ❍ ❍

BP 168/92 his heart muscles are weak

While taking your nursing history, you discover he is in general good health and leads an active life. His current medications include finasteride (Proscar) 5 mg daily and vitamin supplements. He reports that he hasn't been able to void in 12 hours and is very uncomfortable. He asks whether there is anything you can do to help him.

2. During your initial assessment, what finding would you expect in regard to his CC? ❍ ❍ ❍ ❍ ❍

3. What are your nursing priorities for this patient? ❍ ❍ ❍ ❍ ❍

4. After examining M.B., the ED physician asks you to insert a indwelling urinary catheter. What should you include in M.B.'s teaching regarding the placement of an indwelling urinary catheter?

Insertion of the catheter is often painful; in addition, he will feel pressure while the catheter is advanced up the urethra. Once the catheter is in place and urine is drained, he should have a rapid relief of his symptoms.

5. After 2 attempts at placing the catheter you are frustrated because you are unable to advance the catheter without forcing it. What is your next intervention? Why?

After successful placement of the urinary catheter, M.B. reports his bladder feels more comfortable. M.B. informs you he is scheduled for surgery in the coming week because "the doctor told me the pills were not working." M.B.'s urologist calls with the following orders: admit to urology, condition stable; diet as tolerated; NPO after midnight; consent for transurethral resection of the prostate (TURP).

6. What general preoperative teaching would you provide for M.B.?

7. What specific preoperative teaching would you provide regarding a TURP?

Case Study 6

Name ______________________ Class/Group ______ Date ______

Group Members ____

INSTRUCTIONS: All questions apply to this case study. Your responses should be brief and to the point. Adequate space has been provided for answers. When asked to provide several answers, they should be listed in order of priority or significance. Do not assume information that is not provided. Please print or write clearly. If your response is not legible, it will be marked as ? and you will need to rewrite it.

Scenario

You are the nurse in a walk-in clinic. A.P. is being seen this morning for a 2-day history of diffuse but severe abdominal pain. She has c/o nausea without vomiting but denies vaginal bleeding or discharge. A.P. claims to have had unprotected sex with several partners, some of whom have c/o penile discharge. Her last menstrual period ended 3 days ago. She has no known medication allergies and denies previous medical or psychiatric problems. VS are 108/60, 110, 20, 100.6° F (tympanic).

Physical exam finds her abdomen is very tender. The slightest touch of her abdomen causes her to "jump off the exam table." Bowel sounds are normal. Pelvic exam finds purulent material pooled in the vaginal vault, which appears to be coming from the cervix. A sample of the vaginal drainage is obtained and sent for culture.

1. What medical interventions can you anticipate?

2. Based on A.P.'s stated history and the results of the vaginal exam, the physician treats her also for *Chlamydia* infection. Formulate a nursing plan for A.P. that can be shared with the community agency for follow-up.

3. Based on the previous question, identify the potential issues for noncompliance and what other action might encourage successful compliance.

The physician has the option of treating A.P. by one of two different methods. First, the physician could prescribe treatment over a period of 1 week; A.P. would be given the first dose of doxycycline (Monodox) 100 mg PO, then would be given a prescription for the same to be taken PO bid x 7 days. Second, the physician could prescribe a one-time dose of azithromycin (Zithromax) 1 g PO, which could be administered in the clinic.

4. A one-time dose of azithromycin 1 g PO is ordered for A.P. Why is this a good choice for her?

5. *Chlamydia* infection is considered a sexually transmitted disease (STD) that has not been mandated to be reported to the Public Health Department (PHD). Why would the PHD wish to see this become a reportable disease?

6. You ask if someone has talked with A.P. about "safe sex." She laughs and tells you there is nothing safe about sex. Undaunted, you ask if she would be willing for you to discuss the use of condoms with her sexual partners. She tells you that she's already careful; if she doesn't know the guy, she uses condoms every time. How are you going to respond?

7. You ask A.P. if she has been tested for HIV. She says no, she doesn't know anyone with AIDS, and she doesn't do sex with gay men. Now what are you going to say?

8. You ask her if she would like to be tested for HIV. It won't cost her anything, and no one has to know; it's completely confidential. She agrees to the test and it comes back positive. What is her prognosis?

Case Study 7

Name ______________________ Class/Group ______ Date ______

Group Members ____

INSTRUCTIONS: All questions apply to this case study. Your responses should be brief and to the point. Adequate space has been provided for answers. When asked to provide several answers, they should be listed in order of priority or significance. Do not assume information that is not provided. Please print or write clearly. If your response is not legible, it will be marked as ? and you will need to rewrite it.

❍ ❍ ❍ / ❍ ❍

Scenario

S.M. is a 68-year-old man who is being seen at your clinic for routine health maintenance and health promotion. He reports that he has been feeling very well and has no specific complaints except for some trouble "emptying his bladder." He had a CBC and chemistry survey completed 1 week before his visit, and the results are as follows: Na 140 mmol/L, K 4.2 mmol/L, Cl 100 mmol/L, HCO_3 26 mmol/L, BUN 22 mg/dL, creatinine 0.8 mg/dL, glucose 94 mg/dL, RBC 5.2 mil/cmm, WBC 7.4 thou/cmm, Hgb 15.2 g/dL, Hct 46%, platelets 348 thou/cmm. His VS at this visit are 148/88, 82, 16.

1. What can you tell S.M. about his lab work? ❍ ❍ ❍ ❍ ❍

While obtaining your nursing history, you discover that there is no family history of cancer or other genitourinary problems. During further questioning you discover that S.M. has had progressive symptoms over the past 6 months, which include the urge to urinate frequently, decreased ability in starting the stream of urine, and decrease in the force of the urinary steam. The health care provider examines S.M. and reports that his prostate is enlarged and gives a tentative diagnosis of benign prostatic hyperplasia (BPH). The health care provider also orders a clean-catch urine and PSA test.

2. S.M. is curious why this condition would affect his urination. What would you teach him? ❍ ❍ ❍ ❍ ❍

3. Why were the additional tests, UA and PSA, ordered? ❍ ❍ ❍ ❍ ❍

4. What concepts would you include in teaching S.M. to obtain a clean-catch urine specimen for UA?

S.M.'s UA returns with results that are within normal limits (wnl). His PSA is 2.0 ng/mL. The health care provider informs S.M. his blood work was normal. S.M. tells you he still has several questions. What information would you include in answering his following questions?

5. S.M. asks you, "Do I have cancer?"

6. "Will this condition affect my relationship with my wife?" What do you tell him?

7. Before being discharged, the health care provider gives S.M. a prescription for doxazosin with instructions to take 1 mg/d x 7 days, then 2 mg/d x 7 days, and then 4 mg/d thereafter. What type of drug is doxazosin, and what are other indications for the use of this drug?

8. What are the most common side effects for this drug class?

9. From a safety standpoint, what information does S.M. need to know about his treatment with doxazocin?

Case Study 8

Name ____________________ Class/Group ______ Date ______

Group Members ______________________________

INSTRUCTIONS: All questions apply to this case study. Your responses should be brief and to the point. Adequate space has been provided for answers. When asked to provide several answers, they should be listed in order of priority or significance. Do not assume information that is not provided. Please print or write clearly. If your response is not legible, it will be marked as ? and you will need to rewrite it.

Scenario

It is a hot summer day, and you are an afternoon nurse in the ED. S.R., an 18-year-old woman, presents at the ED with severe L flank and abdominal pain, and N/V. S.R. looks very tired, her skin is warm to touch, and she is perspiring. She paces about the room doubled-over and is clutching her abdomen. S.R. tells you that the pain started early this morning and has been pretty steady for 6 hours. Her abdomen is soft and without tenderness, but her L flank is extremely tender to touch/palpation. She is obviously in a great deal of pain. You place S.R. in one of the exam rooms and take the following VS: 138/88, 90, 20, 99° F. Urinalysis shows hematuria. A flat plate x-ray of the abdomen and an intravenous pyelogram (IVP) confirm the diagnosis of a kidney stone low in the L ureter.

S.R.'s mother is in the waiting area and seems to be intoxicated. She is quite noisy, belligerent, and has a strong smell of alcohol. She is obviously upsetting her daughter and is disturbing other patients and their families. The mother is berating you and the other staff members in her loudest voice, "You need to do something, NOW. Don't you know how to do anything?"

1. What is your first priority, and why?

S.R. is seen by a urologist. His plan is to control her pain, prevent infection, and encourage fluids to flush out the stone. She receives a dose of intravenous meperidine (Demerol), which eases her pain for the time being. His orders are as follows: discharge to home, encourage fluids, and strain all urine. Prescriptions include oxycodone (Percocet) 1 or 2 tabs PO q4h for pain and levofloxasin 500 mg PO qd.

2. What specific instructions will you give S.R. about her urine, fluid intake, medications, and activity?

3. What factors may impede S.R.'s comprehension of your instructions, and how can you increase her retention of important information?

4. S.R. is quite young to develop a renal calculi. She may need to understand how she can prevent the development of stones in the future. What factors lead to development of the stones?

5. The urologist schedules S.R. for a follow-up visit in 2 days. He informs her that if the stone has not passed by then, he will schedule her for extracorporeal shock-wave lithotripsy (ESWL). The physician's explanation to S.R. is quite technical and confusing to her. In appropriate terminology, explain to S.R. the concepts and principles of ESWL. ❍ ❍ ❍ ❍ ❍

6. S.R.s' pain has been controlled by the use of narcotics. Her mother is still obviously intoxicated. What ramifications might this have on discharging S.R.? Discuss the issues, and generate several possible actions. ❍ ❍ ❍ ❍ ❍

7. In view of her mother's condition, you are concerned about sending S.R. home with narcotics. How would you discuss this issues with S.R.? ❍ ❍ ❍ ❍ ❍

8. You notice S.R. appears to be embarrassed to discuss her mother with you. How will you respond? ❍ ❍ ❍ ❍ ❍

Case Study 9

Name ______________________ Class/Group ______ Date ______

Group Members ______________________________________

INSTRUCTIONS: All questions apply to this case study. Your responses should be brief and to the point. Adequate space has been provided for answers. When asked to provide several answers, they should be listed in order of priority or significance. Do not assume information that is not provided. Please print or write clearly. If your response is not legible, it will be marked as ? and you will need to rewrite it.

❍ ❍ ❍ / ❍ ❍

Scenario

F.F., a 58-year-old man with type 2 DM (noninsulin-dependent diabetes mellitus), presents at the ED with severe R flank and abdominal pain, and N/V. The abdomen is soft and without tenderness. The right flank is extremely tender to touch and palpation. VS are 142/80, 88, 20, 99.0° F; urinalysis shows hematuria; an IV of .9 NS is started and is to infuse at 125 ml/h. An intravenous pyelogram confirms the diagnosis of a staghorn-type stone in the R renal pelvis. The right kidney looks enlarged. F.F. states that he did not sleep well last night and has not eaten much today. He is obviously very fatigued. His laboratory results are as follows: Na 144 mmol/L, K 4.0 mmol/L, Cl 101 mmol/L, CO_2 26 mmol/L, BUN 30 mg/dL, creatinine 3.6 mg/dL, glucose 260 mg/dL, uric acid 5.0 mg/dL, Ca 9.0 mg/dL, Phos 2.6 mg/dL, total protein 7.8 g/dL, albumin 4.0 g/dL, total-bili 0.3 mg/dL, direct-bili 0.1 mg/dL, Chol 200 mg/dL, Alk phos 61 U/L, LDH total 100 U/L, AST (SGOT) 13 U/L, ALT (SGPT) 13 U/L, GGTP 40 U/L, amylase 98 U/L.

❍ ❍ ❍ ❍ ❍

1. F.F. is treated with IV morphine for pain. It is late afternoon before he is admitted to your unit and scheduled for lithotripsy in the morning. What specific priorities do you identify for F.F.?

2. The physician has prescribed gentamicin 80 mg IVPB q8h. You question the physician about giving this large a dose of gentamicin to F.F. You are met with angry and belittling statements. Articulate why you should question this specific order for F.F.

3. How should you handle the situation with the physician in order to protect the patient and promote a collegial relationship?

4. Hydronephrosis is a potential complication for F.F. What may be the impact of this problem on his long-term kidney function?

5. Analyze the relationship between creatinine and GFR and predicting kidney function.

6. Later, as you walk past his bed, you notice F.F. crawling off the end of the bed. What are you going to do?

F.F. is going to be admitted. You call the unit nurse to give report. You tell her he's been up all night with pain that has just been relieved by IV morphine. You don't know whether he's going to have lithotripsy or surgery; surgery is unlikely because the stone is so large.

7. You tell F.F. he is going to be admitted and will probably need surgery for his kidney stone. He looks at you, panicked, and says, "I can't do that. I don't have any insurance. This is costing me a wad already." How are you going to respond?

❍ ❍ ❍ ❍ ❍

Case Study 10

Name ______________________ Class/Group ______ Date ______

Group Members ____________________________________

INSTRUCTIONS: All questions apply to this case study. Your responses should be brief and to the point. Adequate space has been provided for answers. When asked to provide several answers, they should be listed in order of priority or significance. Do not assume information that is not provided. Please print or write clearly. If your response is not legible, it will be marked as ? and you will need to rewrite it.

Scenario

You are working in the ICU of an acute care hospital and assume the care of E.B., a 78-year-old woman who is 3 days postinferior wall MI. E.B. had been healthy before admission except for a long-standing history of osteoarthritis treated with piroxicam (Feldene) 20 mg daily and severe long-standing hypertension treated with atenolol (Tenormin) 50 mg daily. She also takes omeprazole to prevent NSAID-induced duodenal ulcers. On presentation to the ED, E.B. had severe hypertension (210/122 mm Hg); therefore, thrombolytics were contraindicated and she was taken directly to the cardiac catheterization lab for acute percutaneous transluminal coronary angioplasty (PTCA). Her angioplasty was successful, and she has been pain-free since the PTCA. You are reviewing E.B.'s lab work and note the following values: Na 142 mmol/L, K 4.9 mmol/L, Cl 100 mmol/L, CO_2 26 mmol/L, BUN 28 mg/dL, creatinine 2.2 mg/dL, glucose 158 mg/dL.

1. What abnormalities are there in E.B.'s lab work?

2. What are possible causes for these abnormalities?

3. Describe prerenal, intrarenal, and postrenal causes of acute renal failure (ARF). Given the potential causes of E.B.'s elevated BUN and creatinine, how would they be categorized?

You are given the results of E.B.'s lab work from today. The results are Na 140 mmol/L, K 6.0 mmol/L, Cl 104 mmol/L, CO_2 24 mmol/L, BUN 68 mg/dL, creatinine 4.0 mg/dL, glucose 104 mg/dL. You have also noted her urine output for the past 8 hours is 160 ml.

4. Based on these values, what is your next action going to be?

5. Define *oliguria* and *anuria*. Which term best describes E.B.'s renal function?

6. In reviewing E.B.'s VS, you cannot identify any episodes of hypotension since her admission. What might be a possible explanation for her increase in BUN and creatinine?

7. What are your nursing interventions and priorities for a patient in ARF?

8. E.B. has been very quiet. Suddenly she asks you, "Am I going to die?" How will you respond?

9. You talk to her about the possibility of dialysis, which may be a treatment for her. She responds, "You know, I'm 78 years old. I've had a pretty good life and I don't want to be hooked to a machine." What will you say?

Case Study 11

Name ______________________ Class/Group ______ Date ______

Group Members ______________________________________

INSTRUCTIONS: All questions apply to this case study. Your responses should be brief and to the point. Adequate space has been provided for answers. When asked to provide several answers, they should be listed in order of priority or significance. Do not assume information that is not provided. Please print or write clearly. If your response is not legible, it will be marked as ? and you will need to rewrite it.

Scenario

M.Z., an 89-year-old widow, recently experienced a left cerebrovascular accident (CVA). She has R-sided weakness and expressive aphasia with swallowing difficulty. M.Z. has a PMH of L CVA 2.5 years previous, chronic atrial flutter, and hypertension. M.Z. has a negative psychiatric history and has lived with her daughter's family in a rural town since her previous stroke. Since admission to an acute care facility 5 days ago, M.Z. has gained some strength, has become oriented to person and place, and is anxious to begin her rehabilitation program. M.Z. is transferred for rehabilitation to your skilled nursing facility with the following orders: hydrochlorothiazide 25 mg PO qd, digoxin 0.125 mg PO qd, aspirin 81 mg PO qd, warfarin (Coumadin) 5 mg PO qd, Tylenol 325 mg q6h prn for pain, zolpidem 5 mg PO hs prn for sleep. Diet: mechanical soft, low Na with ground meat. Other strategies: maintain Foley to DD and then follow up with bladder training; facilitate referrals for speech, OT, and PT to evaluate and treat swallowing, communication, and functional abilities.

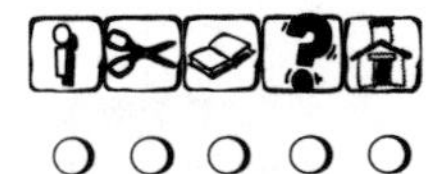

1. What lab orders would you anticipate as a result of this specific list of orders? With each response, describe your rationale.

2. At the interdisciplinary care conferences, you report that bladder training is progressing and recommend removing the catheter if M.Z.'s mobility and communication abilities have progressed sufficiently. The group and M.Z. agree that she is ready for the Foley to be removed. Identify three problems that M.Z. is at risk for developing following catheter removal. Describe specific nursing interventions for each problem.

3. Two days after the Foley is removed, you observe that M.Z.'s urine is cloudy and concentrated and has a strong odor. What are your immediate actions?

4. M.Z. is started on sulfamethoxazole 400 mg/trimethoprim 160 mg (Bactrim DS) 1 tab PO bid x 10 days. However, 2 days later you find M.Z. in the bathroom on the toilet, and she is very upset. There is blood on the floor next to the toilet, and the water is bright red with clots. You help her clean herself, help her into bed, and provide emotional support. Describe your assessment steps. What complications do you anticipate?

5. You complete your assessment and report your findings to the physician. You obtain an order for a straight catheterized specimen for C&S. Identify at least 2 causes for M.Z.'s hematuria.

6. M.Z.'s UTI is responding to antibiotics, and you want to prepare M.Z. and her daughter for eventual discharge. What specific issues must be considered in the teaching/discharge planning to prevent a recurrence of infection?

7. You talk with M.Z.'s daughter about her understanding of caregiving responsibilities for her mother. What kind of questions are you going to ask to assess if she is capable of taking on this additional burden?

Case Study 12

Name ______________________________ Class/Group ______ Date ______

Group Members ____

INSTRUCTIONS: All questions apply to this case study. Your responses should be brief and to the point. Adequate space has been provided for answers. When asked to provide several answers, they should be listed in order of priority or significance. Do not assume information that is not provided. Please print or write clearly. If your response is not legible, it will be marked as ? and you will need to rewrite it.

❍ ❍ ❍ / ❍ ❍

Scenario

T.C. is a 30-year-old woman who three weeks ago underwent a vaginal hysterectomy, right salpingo-oophorectomy for abdominal pain, and endometriosis. Postoperatively she experienced an intraabdominal hemorrhage, and her Hct dropped from 40.5% to 21%. She was transfused with 3 units of RBCs. Following discharge she continued to have abdominal pain, chills, and fever and was subsequently readmitted twice: once for treatment of postop infection and the second time for evacuation of pelvic hematoma. Despite treatment, T.C. continued to have abdominal pain, chills, fever, and N/V.

T.C. has now been admitted to your unit following an exploratory laparotomy. VS are 130/70, 94, 16, 37.6° F (tympanic). She is easily aroused and oriented to place and person. She dozes between verbal requests. She has a low-midline abdominal dressing that is dry and intact and a Jackson-Pratt (JP) drain that is fully compressed and contains a scant amount of bright red blood. Her Foley to down drain has clear yellow urine. She has an IV of 1000 ml $D_5{}^1\!/_2$NS infusing at 100 ml/h in her L forearm, with no swelling or redness. T.C. is receiving IV morphine sulfate for pain control through a patient-controlled analgesia (PCA) pump. The settings are dose 2 mg, lock-out interval 15 min, 4 hour max of 30 mg. When aroused, she states that her pain is an 8 on a scale of 1 to 10. She also has 2 L O_2/nc, and her SaO_2 by pulse oximeter is 93%.

❍ ❍ ❍ ❍ ❍

1. During your assessment, you note that T.C.'s R is 16 and shallow. Articulate your plan for a more complete assessment of T.C.s' condition. Include factors to be considered, the supporting rationale, and your nursing actions.

The unit is very busy when T.C. is returned from the postanesthesia care unit (PACU). Staffing is minimal. You are concerned about monitoring T.C. carefully enough. Your present patient load is 6; of those, 2 patients are newly postop and 1 is getting ready for discharge. You have a nursing assistant who helps you and another R.N. You are most concerned with T.C.'s respiratory status and the possibility that she may, in her drowsy state, self-administer a dose of narcotic that would further reduce her respiratory status.

2. Formulate a plan, given the resources mentioned previously. ❍ ❍ ❍ ❍ ❍

3. Pain control using the PCA can be very tricky. Throughout the first postop day, it has been difficult to juggle T.C.'s need for pain medication and depression of her respiratory status. Discuss the concepts of controlling pain with IV narcotics and factors that may be adjusted to better control her pain. ❍ ❍ ❍ ❍ ❍

4. T.C. is beginning to withdraw from conversations with you and the other staff. She sleeps most of the day and is not eating. At times she is tearful and is irritable with her husband. You believe that she is showing signs of depression. What actions should you take to help her? ❍ ❍ ❍ ❍ ❍

5. T.C. and her husband are talking one evening, and you overhear that they are very dissatisfied with the care provided by the physician. They believe that he has mismanaged T.C.'s care. They are discussing getting an attorney. They ask you what you think. What do you do?

6. You state, "Tell me what's going on with you right now. Maybe I can help you be more comfortable." What would be the benefit of taking this approach?

7. Mr. C. says, "No one is telling us anything. My wife came in here for a simple hysterectomy, she ends up with 4 surgeries, she still has pain, and she's worse off than when she started. Somebody has screwed up big time. Then they have the nerve to send me a bill. This morning they demanded $185,000. I'm not paying a dime until she gets better." How are you going to respond?

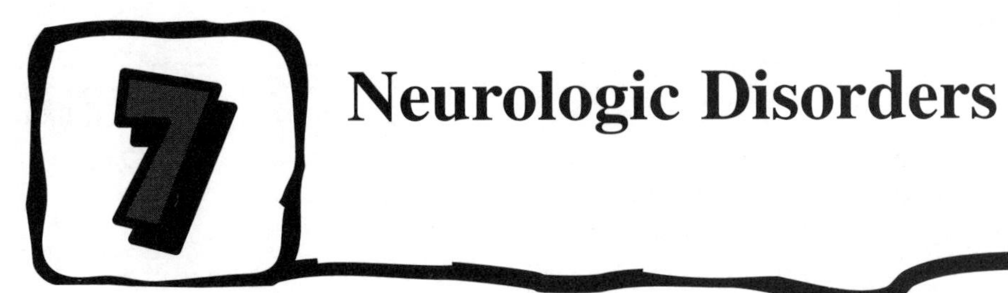

Neurologic Disorders

Case Study 1

Name ______________________ Class/Group ______ Date ______

Group Members ______________________________________

INSTRUCTIONS: All questions apply to this case study. Your responses should be brief and to the point. Adequate space has been provided for answers. When asked to provide several answers, they should be listed in order of priority or significance. Do not assume information that is not provided. Please print or write clearly. If your response is not legible, it will be marked as ? and you will need to rewrite it.

Scenario

M.E. is a 62-year-old woman who has a 5-year history of progressive forgetfulness. She is no longer able to care for herself, has becomes increasingly depressed and paranoid, and recently started a fire in the kitchen. After extensive neurologic evaluation, M.E. was diagnosed as having Alzheimer's disease. Her husband and children have come to the Alzheimer's unit at your extended-care facility (ECF) for information about this disease and to discuss the possibility of placement for M.E. You reassure the family that you have experience dealing with questions and concerns most people in their situation have.

1. How would you explain Alzheimer's disease to the family?

2. The husband asks, "How did she get Alzheimer's? We don't know anyone else who has it." How would you respond?

3. After asking the family to describe M.E.'s behavior, you determine that she is in stage 2 of Alzheimer's 3 stages. Describe common s/s for each stage of the disease.

4. The daughter expresses frustration at the number of tests M.E. had to undergo and the length of time it took for someone to diagnosis M.E.'s problem. What tests are likely to be performed and how is Alzheimer's disease diagnosed?

The husband states, "How are you going to take care of her? She wanders around all night long. She can't find her way to the bathroom in a house she's lived in for 43 years. She can't be trusted to be alone any more; she almost burnt the house down. We're all exhausted; there are three of us, and we can't keep up with her. "You acknowledge how exhausted they must be from trying to keep her safe. You tell the family that there is no known treatment and that Alzheimer's units have been created to provide a structured, safe environment for each person."

5. Describe the Alzheimer's-related nursing interventions r/t each of the following nursing care problems: self-care deficits, disturbed sleep pattern, impaired verbal communication, impaired cognitive function, risk for injury. ❍ ❍ ❍ ❍ ❍

6. M.E.'s son asks what different medications might be prescribed for M.E. How would you describe the purpose of antiseizure, cognitive, antipsychotic, antidepressive, or sedative medications for a patient like M.E.? ❍ ❍ ❍ ❍ ❍

You try to comfort the family by telling them that the problems they are experiencing are very common. You explain that family support is a major focus of your program.

7. List four ways that M.E.'s family might receive the support they need.

Select and print out at least one professional-quality Internet resource for research information on Alzheimer's:

- *http://www.nih.gov/health/* is an authoritative reference for general health information on nearly any subject. Most Alzheimer's research is conducted by the National Institute of Neurological Disorders and Stroke (NINDS).
- *http://www.ninds.nih.gov/* has information for the public, health care professionals (clinicians), and scientists (researchers). Many NIH resources also have public information available in Spanish.
- Another important reference is the Alzheimer's Disease Education and Referral (ADEAR) Center (*http://www.alzheimers.org/*), a service of the National Institute on Aging (*http://www.nih.gov/nia/*).
- General Information:
    - Patients and families who are dealing with incurable disorders are often victimized by opportunists who offer treatments that are not scientifically based. Sometimes these treatments may even be dangerous. Two valuable resources for checking on the value of alternative treatments or identifying "quack" cures are:
        - *http://www.quackwatch.com/*
        - *http://nccam.nih.gov/* (National Center for Complementary and Alternative Medicine)

Case Study 2

Name ______________________ Class/Group ______ Date ______

Group Members ______________________________________

INSTRUCTIONS: All questions apply to this case study. Your responses should be brief and to the point. Adequate space has been provided for answers. When asked to provide several answers, they should be listed in order of priority or significance. Do not assume information that is not provided. Please print or write clearly. If your response is not legible, it will be marked as ? and you will need to rewrite it.

Scenario

D.S. is a 74-year-old retired social worker who has been on your floor for several days receiving q.o.d. plasmapheresis for myasthenia gravis (MG). She has a PMH of type 2 DM for 3 years and low back pain secondary to spinal stenosis. She received 2 steroid injections into her spine for pain 2 to 3 weeks before her admission, which was followed by progressive, symmetric, weakness in her lower extremities proximal > distal; R foot numbness; poor eye-hand coordination; and significant hand weakness. On admission, D.S. was unable to bear any weight or take fluids through a straw. There have been periods of exacerbation and remission since admission.

1. You are visiting with D.S.'s grandson who tells you he is just starting medical school and he would like to know more about MG so that he can discuss it with his grandmother. What do you tell him?

2. He asks you to explain how plasmapheresis works. How would you explain this treatment?

3. He asks what drugs are used to treat MG. You explain that although neostigmine (Prostigmin) and pyridostigmine (Mestinon) are often used in combination, drug regimens and doses are highly individualized. Identify the appropriate drug classification and explain the action of these two drugs to D.S.'s grandson.

4. D.S. told her grandson that after taking her morning medications, she often experienced nausea, heartburn, slight SOB, sweating, and she felt her heart beating rapidly. What can you tell him about this?

5. Describe a myasthenic crisis.

6. List six nursing problem statements that would be appropriate for D.S.

7. List five factors that could predispose D.S. to an exacerbation of her illness.

8. D.S. asks you what the doctors meant when they were talking about some kind of a challenge test. You realize they must have been discussing the possibility of performing an edrophonium (Tensilon) challenge. What is a Tensilon challenge, and what information will it yield?

9. What are aminoglycosides, and why are they contraindicated in patients with MG?

10. D.S.'s grandson wants to know when she'll be able to go home. How do you respond?

11. What supportive measures can you suggest to D.S.'s grandson that he can undertake or arrange on behalf of his grandmother?

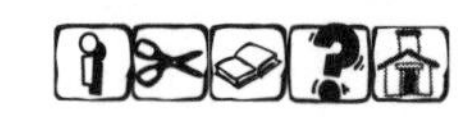

❍ ❍ ❍ ❍ ❍

Bonus Question: Which institute under the National Institutes of Health is primarily responsible for myasthenia gravis information and research?

Note: Another excellent source of information is:

Myasthenia Gravis Foundation of America
123 W. Madison Street
Suite 800
Chicago, IL 60602
Telephone: (800) 541-5454 Fax: (312) 853-0523
E-mail: info-request@myasthenia.org

Case Study 3

Name ______________ Class/Group ______ Date ______

Group Members ______________

INSTRUCTIONS: All questions apply to this case study. Your responses should be brief and to the point. Adequate space has been provided for answers. When asked to provide several answers, they should be listed in order of priority or significance. Do not assume information that is not provided. Please print or write clearly. If your response is not legible, it will be marked as ? and you will need to rewrite it.

Scenario

J.G. is a 34-year-old P1 G1 woman who underwent an emergency cesarean delivery after a prolonged labor, during which she exhibited a sudden change in neurologic functioning and started seizing. Since that time, she has experienced 3 tonic-clonic (grand mal) seizures. She was diagnosed as having a basal ganglion hematoma with infarct and was started on phenytoin. Postdelivery, J.G. demonstrated dyskinesia, resulting in frequent falls during ambulation. Once the seizure disorder appeared to be under control, she was transferred to a rehabilitation facility for evaluation, and 2 weeks of intensive PT. She is now home, where she is doing quite well but still has occasional falls and is receiving PT 3 times a week in her home. She remains on phenytoin and has had no seizures since her release from the rehabilitation facility. As case manager for J.G.'s HMO, you visit her and her family at home for evaluation of long-term, follow-up care.

1. A seizure is not a disease in itself but a symptom of a disease. What is the term for chronically recurring seizures?

   EPILEPSY

2. Does J.G. have epilepsy?

3. The 3 main phases of a seizure are the preictal, ictal, and postictal. Differentiate between the 3 phases, and list clinical symptoms you may observe when a patient is having a seizure.

4. What is the pathophysiology of a seizure?

5. J.G. had grand mal, or tonic-clonic, seizures. Describe this type of seizure. List five other types of seizures. ❍ ❍ ❍ ❍ ❍

6. Some patients know they are about to have a seizure. What is this preseizure warning called, and what form does it take? ❍ ❍ ❍ ❍ ❍

7. Besides the brain injury, what are some other possible conditions that could be contributing to J.G's lowered seizure threshold? ❍ ❍ ❍ ❍ ❍

8. List five different classifications of antiseizure medications. ❍ ❍ ❍ ❍ ❍

9. J.G.'s husband comes to visit and asks you what he should do if she has a seizure at home. What would do you tell him? ❍ ❍ ❍ ❍ ❍

10. Her husband states that he is afraid for J.G. to take care of the baby. What would you say to him? ❍ ❍ ❍ ❍ ❍

11. J.G.'s husband tells you that his wife is not good at remembering to take medication. What are some strategies that you should review with J.G. and her husband to increase the likelihood of compliance? ❍ ❍ ❍ ❍ ❍

12. J.G. asks, "If I get my blood level under control, will it stay at the same level as long as I take my medicine?" How would you answer her question? ❍ ❍ ❍ ❍ ❍

13. J.G.'s husband asks whether the drugs could harm his wife in any way. What general information would you give them about anticonvulsants? ❍ ❍ ❍ ❍ ❍

14. J.G.'s husband says, "I was watching *Emergency* last night, and they showed this guy who just kept on having a seizure. That doctor had to give him lots of medicine before he came out of it." How would you explain status epilepticus, and why is it a medical emergency? ❍ ❍ ❍ ❍ ❍

Optional Project: Look up the MedicAlert Web site, and plan a 10-minute presentation for patients/consumers/families on the importance of people with seizure disorders wearing standardized identification. Include instructions on cost, benefits, and how they can get MedicAlert identification.

For additional information contact:

MedicAlert
2323 Colorado Avenue
Turlock, CA 95382
Telephone: (800) 432-5378
Website: *http://www.medicalert.org*

Case Study 4

Name ______________________ Class/Group ______ Date ______

Group Members ____

INSTRUCTIONS: All questions apply to this case study. Your responses should be brief and to the point. Adequate space has been provided for answers. When asked to provide several answers, they should be listed in order of priority or significance. Do not assume information that is not provided. Please print or write clearly. If your response is not legible, it will be marked as ? and you will need to rewrite it.

Scenario

You have been asked to see D.V. in the neurologic clinic. D.V. has been referred by his internist, who thinks his patient is having symptoms of multiple sclerosis (MS). D.V. is a 20-year-old man who has experienced increasing urinary frequency and urgency over the past 2 months. Because his female partner was treated for an STD, D.V. also underwent treatment, but the symptoms did not resolve. D.V. has also recently had 2 brief episodes of eye "fuzziness" associated with diplopia and brightness. He has noticed ascending numbness and weakness of the R arm with inability to hold objects over the past few days. Now he reports rapid progression of weakness in his legs.

1. MS is an inflammatory disorder of the nervous system causing scattered, patchy demyelinization of the CNS. What does myelin do? What is demyelinization?

2. MS is characterized by remissions and exacerbations. What happens to the myelin during each of these phases?

3. Isn't D.V. too young to get MS? What is the etiology?

4. What assessment data from the case study caused the physician to suspect a possible diagnosis of MS?

Diagnostic tests are often done to R/O other disorders with similar symptoms. A diagnosis will be made when other disorders have been R/O, when the patient has 2 or more exacerbations, when there is slow, steady progression, and/or when the patient has 2 or more areas of demyelinization or plaque formation.

5. What are four common diagnostic tests you can begin to teach D.V. about? ❍ ❍ ❍ ❍ ❍

6. D.V. asks you, "If this turns out to be MS, what is the treatment?" ❍ ❍ ❍ ❍ ❍

7. As part of your teaching plan, you want D.V. to be aware of situations or factors that are known to cause an exacerbation of symptoms. List four. ❍ ❍ ❍ ❍ ❍

8. The National Multiple Sclerosis Society, 733 3rd Ave., 6th Floor, New York, NY 10017-3288 (800-344-4867), is a great resource for D.V. List several resources available in the community that D.V. may find helpful. ❍ ❍ ❍ ❍ ❍

D.V. confides in you that he tried to commit suicide at the age of 14 when his parents got a divorce. He tells you that he knows his girlfriend hasn't been faithful, but he's afraid of living alone. He admits that she occasionally hits him, but he's afraid if he tells her about his M.S. diagnosis, she'll leave him for good. You recall seeing yellowish bruises on his arms when you took his admission BP.

9. What are you going to do with this information? ❍ ❍ ❍ ❍ ❍

10. In view of his personal history and current diagnosis, what two critical psychosocial issues are you going to monitor for in his follow-up visits? ❍ ❍ ❍ ❍ ❍

D.V. takes advantage of his time with the psychiatric nurse specialist, joins a local MS support group, and tells his girlfriend to move out. He later marries a woman from the support group.

Case Study 5

Name ______________________ Class/Group ______ Date ______

Group Members ____

INSTRUCTIONS: All questions apply to this case study. Your responses should be brief and to the point. Adequate space has been provided for answers. When asked to provide several answers, they should be listed in order of priority or significance. Do not assume information that is not provided. Please print or write clearly. If your response is not legible, it will be marked as ? and you will need to rewrite it.

❍ ❍ ❍ / ❍ ❍

Scenario

S.B. is a 28-year-old married woman with a PMH of seizure disorder controlled with Tegretol (last seizure was 5 years ago), hypothyroidism controlled with Synthroid, and a recent URI. On a day outing with her family, she slipped and fell, landing on the back of her head. She experienced loss of consciousness at the scene. She was taken to a local hospital where a CT scan revealed a L subdural hematoma. She has been transferred to your regional medical center, which has a neurosurgeon on call.

1. The ED RN gives you the above information during a phoned report. What other information do you need to prepare for this patient? ❍ ❍ ❍ ❍ ❍

2. Because you always have trouble remembering the layers of the brain and different hematomas, you look up subdural hematoma before S.B. arrives. What do you find? ❍ ❍ ❍ ❍ ❍

3. S.B.'s subdural is considered acute because symptoms appeared within 24 hours of injury. What are the other classifications of subdural hematomas? ❍ ❍ ❍ ❍ ❍

4. What are common s/s of an acute subdural hematoma? ❍ ❍ ❍ ❍ ❍

5. Why are the elderly and alcoholics at risk for chronic subdural hematomas? ❍ ❍ ❍ ❍ ❍

6. How would you monitor for neurologic change? ❍ ❍ ❍ ❍ ❍

7. Why is it especially important to make sure S.B. is taking her tegretal and has a therapeutic serum level? ❍ ❍ ❍ ❍ ❍

8. The decision was made in S.B.'s case not to do a craniotomy. When would a neurosurgeon decide to treat medically vs. perform surgery? ❍ ❍ ❍ ❍ ❍

9. Burr holes work only for acute subdurals, and a craniotomy must be done for subacute and chronic subdurals. Why? ❍ ❍ ❍ ❍ ❍

10. Why would hypotonic IV solutions such as D_5W be avoided? ❍ ❍ ❍ ❍ ❍

11. How would you position S.B. in bed? ❍ ❍ ❍ ❍ ❍

12. If S.B.'s LOC started to decrease, what information would you give the neurosurgeon when you call?

13. How would you provide support to the family?

14. The neurosurgeon has ordered codeine IV as a pain medication. Why did he order codeine?

Case Study 6

Name ____________________ Class/Group ______ Date ______

Group Members ______________________________

INSTRUCTIONS: All questions apply to this case study. Your responses should be brief and to the point. Adequate space has been provided for answers. When asked to provide several answers, they should be listed in order of priority or significance. Do not assume information that is not provided. Please print or write clearly. If your response is not legible, it will be marked as ? and you will need to rewrite it.

❍ ❍ ❍ / ❍ ❍

Scenario

You are assigned to take care of M.X. this evening's shift. In report you are told that she is a 40-year-old obese (112 kg) woman who arose from a sitting position and experienced acute and severe low back pain 3 weeks ago. She was diagnosed with herniated disks L4-L5 and L5-S1. Dr. W., who performed a lumbar laminectomy 3 days ago, is concerned because her WBC count has gone from 8.1 thou/cmm to 19.6 thou/cmm.

1. What is meant by the term *herniated disk (herniated nucleus pulposus)*? ❍ ❍ ❍ ❍ ❍

2. What tests may be performed to detect and diagnose the herniation? ❍ ❍ ❍ ❍ ❍

3. What is a laminectomy? ❍ ❍ ❍ ❍ ❍

4. Identify two general objectives of postoperative nursing care of M.X.? ❍ ❍ ❍ ❍ ❍

5. What is meant by "log-rolling?" ❍ ❍ ❍ ❍ ❍

6. You ask 4 coworkers to help you log-roll M.X. As one nurse enters the room she makes a statement about breaking her back trying to move M.X. You are a little overweight yourself and watch M.X.'s face when she hears the remark. How would you handle the situation? ❍ ❍ ❍ ❍ ❍

7. Patients who have undergone a lumbar laminectomy frequently experience paralytic ileus and urinary retention. Why? ❍ ❍ ❍ ❍ ❍

8. What are four possible sources of infection that may account for M.X.'s elevated WBC? ❍ ❍ ❍ ❍ ❍

9. M.X. asks you how you would know if her wound were infected. Differentiate between s/s of wound infection for M.X. ❍ ❍ ❍ ❍ ❍

10. Discharge planning should begin the day M.X. is admitted to your unit. What factors should discharge planning include? ❍ ❍ ❍ ❍ ❍

11. List seven written home care instructions that should be reviewed and given to M.X. before discharge. ❍ ❍ ❍ ❍ ❍

M.X. is treated with aggressive antibiotic therapy for a UTI. With the help and support of her family, she is discharged to home where she makes a complete recovery. After referral for consultation with a medical nutritionist, M.X. starts on a healthy low-fat diet and loses 21 pounds over the next 9 months. When you were arranging her discharge papers, you discovered that M.X. was a script writer for soap operas. Six months after her discharge, she calls to meet you for coffee. She asks whether you would like to supplement your income by consulting with her on realistically presenting the role of nurses in soap operas. She said it was your professionalism that gave her this idea.

Case Study 7

Name ______________________ Class/Group ______ Date ______

Group Members ______________________________________

INSTRUCTIONS: All questions apply to this case study. Your responses should be brief and to the point. Adequate space has been provided for answers. When asked to provide several answers, they should be listed in order of priority or significance. Do not assume information that is not provided. Please print or write clearly. If your response is not legible, it will be marked as ? and you will need to rewrite it.

Scenario

F.N. is a 57-year-old housewife, happily married with grown children, and 2 new grandchildren. F.N. made an appointment with her optometrist to explore a progressive OS visual loss over a 9-month period. Her eye exam was essentially normal, and the optometrist referred her to a neurologist. After workup, a 2.5 cm brain mass was found, and surgery was scheduled. Her only past medical history (PMH) is hypertension, for which she takes nifedipine XL 60 mg qd. Her past surgical history (PSH) includes T&A as a child, cholecystectomy, and a TAH at age 42. She also takes a conjugated estrogen (Premarin) 0.625 mg qd.

1. Name four tests that can be done to evaluate for brain tumor.

There is no standardized, universally accepted system of classifying brain tumors. They can be classified according to histologic basis, intraaxial vs. extraaxial, or malignant vs. benign.

2. Using the term *benign* when discussing brain tumors is somewhat misleading. Why?

3. Onset of neurologic symptoms is usually insidious, and they exhibit symptoms in relation to the area of the brain where the tumor is located. List six general symptoms associated with many brain tumors.

4. Dexamethasone (Decadron) is commonly prescribed when a tumor is diagnosed and the presence of IICP is demonstrated. It is administered preoperatively and postoperatively, and in conjunction with radiation and chemotherapy. Why is Decadron prescribed, and why should it not be abruptly stopped?

5. Other common supportive medications include antiseizure, diuretics, H_2 blockers, analgesics, antiemetics, and antidepressants. Indicate why each is used.

6. Once the diagnosis is made, the patient and family must be involved in the plan for treatment. Treatment depends on the type and location of the tumor and can include surgery, radiation, chemotherapy, or any combination of these. The patient also has the right to refuse treatment. Identify four other considerations the medical team, patient, and family will consider in devising a treatment plan.

7. Describe common responses to a diagnosis of a brain tumor.

8. List two nursing problems r/t F.N.'s role/relationships.

9. F.N. draws up a living will and health care power of attorney after she hears the diagnosis. She also sits down with her family and makes her wishes known. Why is this important for F.N. in particular and for everyone in general?

10. You enter F.N.'s room to take VS and she says, "What if I come out of surgery and I'm different? Or what if I die? My grandbabies will never know me." You hear the concern in her voice. Suggest several ways that F.N. can communicate with her loved ones in the event that her surgery is unsuccessful.

11. F.N. has the surgery and is admitted to ICU postop. She does very well and remains neurologically intact (q1h neuro checks). Her BP is slightly elevated (147/68); the rest of her VS are normal; she has 2 peripheral IVs, TED hose, O_2 at 4 L/nc, and a Foley. Postoperatively, F.N.'s K level drops to 2.7 mmol/L, and glucose is 202 mg/dL. Describe possible reasons why these two laboratory values are abnormal, and identify what treatment will be ordered to correct each.

F.N. did suffer mild neurologic damage as a result of the surgery. She was discharged to a rehabilitation facility, and eventually recovered most of her lost function. She continues to enjoy an active life and has become involved in helping others facing similar experiences.

For additional information contact:

The Brain Injury Association Inc.
105 North Alfred Street
Alexandria, VA 22314
Telephone: (703) 236-6000
Fax: (703) 236-6001

Case Study 8

Name ______________________ Class/Group ______ Date ______

Group Members ______________________________________

INSTRUCTIONS: All questions apply to this case study. Your responses should be brief and to the point. Adequate space has been provided for answers. When asked to provide several answers, they should be listed in order of priority or significance. Do not assume information that is not provided. Please print or write clearly. If your response is not legible, it will be marked as ? and you will need to rewrite it.

Scenario

You are working at a skilled nursing facility that cares for patients on ventilators. G.W. is your first patient with Guillain-Barré syndrome. G.W. is a divorced, self-supporting 56-year-old woman from a small town who developed a URI after caring for her grandson who had the same. Three weeks later she developed weakness, numbness, and tingling in her feet that progressed up her body. Her physician recognized the seriousness of her condition and transferred her to a tertiary referral center. Within days she became totally paralyzed; she was trached and placed on mechanical ventilation. She spent 1 month in the neuro critical care unit and several months on the floor before being transferred to your facility. Her only inhospital complication was pneumonia, which has totally resolved. The physicians don't know how long the paralysis will last.

1. What adaptations would you or your family have to make if you were paralyzed and unable to perform your normal responsibilities? How would you feel if you were totally dependent on others for your simplest needs? Use a separate sheet of paper for a detailed response, and include daily care; financial issues, such as who would pay the rent/mortgage, groceries, utilities, mounting medical bills; social issues, such as who would care for your children, see to their education, meet their emotional needs; self-perception; emotions; etc.

2. Is G.W.'s case typical?

3. Why does potentially fatal respiratory dysfunction occur?

4. Describe a plan for pulmonary hygiene for G.W.

5. How do you anticipate that G.W.'s nutritional needs are being met?

6. Describe nursing interventions to manage bladder and bowel elimination for G.W.

7. What are some things you can do to decrease G.W.'s fear and anxiety?

8. You are using your expert nursing skills to avoid complications. List four potential complications.

9. What measures can be taken to prevent pressure ulcers?

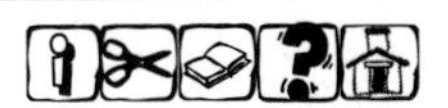

An additional 3 weeks have passed. G.W. has recovered gross movement of her arms and some respiratory effort. She is still on a ventilator, but she has gone from controlled to assisted breathing. This morning G.W. receives a letter from her health insurance company informing her that she has exceeded her lifetime limit and has been dropped from their plan. She is crying hysterically and is choking because of the increased mucous production in her sinuses. Remember that she cannot wipe her eyes or blow her nose to clear it.

10. What can be done for her? ❍ ❍ ❍ ❍ ❍

It takes G.W. almost 11 months to recover enough to be discharged to home with the assistance of a home health aide.

Case Study 9

Name ______________________ Class/Group ______ Date ______

Group Members ____________________________________

INSTRUCTIONS: All questions apply to this case study. Your responses should be brief and to the point. Adequate space has been provided for answers. When asked to provide several answers, they should be listed in order of priority or significance. Do not assume information that is not provided. Please print or write clearly. If your response is not legible, it will be marked as ? and you will need to rewrite it.

Scenario

T.W. is a 22-year-old man who fell 50 feet from a chairlift while skiing and landed on hard-packed snow. He was found to have a T10-11 fracture with paraplegia. He was initially admitted to the SICU and placed on high-dose steroids for 24 hours. He was taken to surgery 48 hours postaccident for spinal stabilization. He spent 2 additional days in the SICU, 5 days on the neuro unit, and now is ready to be transferred to your rehab unit. He continues to have no movement of his lower extremities.

1. The goal of treatment in the acute phase of spinal cord injury (SCI) is to help T.W. survive the injury and maintain physiologic stability through the period of spinal shock. Once the acute phase is over, T.W. moves into the postacute and early rehab phases. What are the treatment goals for T.W. in these phases?

2. Considering a hierarchy of rehabilitative needs for patients like T.W., number the following from highest (1) to lowest (5) priority.

   ___ Community integration and employment
   ___ Accomplishment of self-care and ADLs
   ___ Self-actualization
   ___ Stabilization of the physiologic systems
   ___ Adjustment to living at home

3. T.W. receives high-dose steroid therapy every 24 hours; then he is placed on a smaller maintenance dose. What effect will steroids have on T.W.?

4. List three critical potential infections that T.W. should be monitored for throughout his hospitalization.

A person with an SCI at the T2–12 level should be independent in a wheelchair and able to manage ADLs, including bowel and bladder care.

5. T.W. is taking vitamin C 250 mg PO bid. What is the purpose of this?

You request a consultation with an RD because you realize that T.W. needs proteins for healing; however, too much can stress his kidneys. The RD will adjust his diet to ensure adequate amount of protein, carbohydrates, calcium, magnesium, and zinc.

6. Rehabilitation teaching includes teaching T.W. how to manage his urinary drainage system. What would this teaching include?

7. What is the usual amount of time for the return of reflex function of the bladder?

8. The large bowel musculature has its own neural center that can directly respond to distention caused by fecal material. This is what allows most SCI patients to regain bowel control. What dietary instructions are important for T.W.?

9. T.W. should also be taught bowel training techniques. What would this teaching include?

10. What medications can assist with a bowel program?

11. Describe digital stimulation.

12. T.W. asks you whether he'll ever be able to have sex again. What do you tell him, and what are some possible referrals?

For patients with lesions at T_6 or above, there is the potential for autonomic dysreflexia (AD) in response to noxious stimulation of the sympathetic nervous system. The patient develops severe hypertension (as high as 240–300/150 mm Hg), pounding headache, bradycardia, blurred vision, nausea, nasal congestion, and flushing and sweating above the level of the injury and goose bumps or pallor below the level of the injury. Potential causes include bladder distention, obstruction, infection, spasms, catheterization, and bladder irrigations done too fast or with cold fluid; bowel constipation, impaction, or rectal stimulation; and alterations in skin integrity including pressure, infection, injury, and cold or hot. This can cause retinal hemorrhage, CVA, and seizure activity.

13. What are nursing interventions r/t AD?

For additional information, contact:
National Spinal Cord Injury Association
Telephone: (800) 962-9629
E-mail: *resource@spinalcord.org*

Case Study 10

Name ______________________ Class/Group ______ Date ______

Group Members ____

INSTRUCTIONS: All questions apply to this case study. Your responses should be brief and to the point. Adequate space has been provided for answers. When asked to provide several answers, they should be listed in order of priority or significance. Do not assume information that is not provided. Please print or write clearly. If your response is not legible, it will be marked as ? and you will need to rewrite it.

Scenario

Y.W. is a 23-year-old male student from Thailand studying electrical engineering at the university. He was ejected from a moving vehicle, which was traveling 70 mph. His injuries included a severe closed head injury with an occipital hematoma, bilateral wrist fractures, and a R pneumothorax. During his NICU stay, Y.W. was intubated and placed on mechanical ventilation, had a feeding tube inserted and was placed on tube feedings, had a Foley catheter to down drain, and had multiple IVs inserted. He developed pneumonia 1 month after admission.

1. Describe the term *primary head injury*.

2. Describe secondary head injury.

3. Why is IICP so clinically important, and what are five s/s?

4. List four medication classifications and eight nursing measures that the ICU nurses could use to control or decrease the ICP.

5. Y.W.'s medication list includes clindamycin 150 mg per feeding tube q6h, ranitidine (Zantac elixir) 150 mg per feeding tube bid, and phenytoin (Dilantin) 100 mg IVPB tid. Indicate why he is on each.

6. A STAT portable CXR is ordered after each central venous catheter (CVC) is inserted. According to hospital protocol, no one is permitted to infuse anything through the catheter until the CXR has been read by the physician or radiologist. What is the purpose of the CXR, and why isn't fluid infused through the catheter until after the CXR is read?

Y.W. spent 2 months in acute care and is now on your rehab unit. He follows commands but tends to get very agitated with too much stimulation. His trach site is well healed, and the pneumonia is finally resolving. He is still receiving supplemental tube feeding and has some continued incontinence of both bowel and bladder. Y.W. has a very supportive group of friends who are students at the university; several of them are also from Thailand.

7. Y.W.'s latest lab results are as follows: Na 149 mmol/L, K 4.2 mmol/L, Cl 119 mmol/L, CO_2 21 mmol/L, BUN 12 mg/dL, creatinine 1.2 mg/dL, glucose 123 mg/dL, WBC 15.4 thou/cmm, Hgb 14.9 g/dL, Hct 36.4%, platelets 140 thou/cmm. Are any of these of concern to you, and what would you suggest to correct them? ❍ ❍ ❍ ❍ ❍

8. Are you surprised by Y.W.'s agitated behavior? Explain. ❍ ❍ ❍ ❍ ❍

9. Outline a general rehabilitation plan for Y.W. based on the above data. ❍ ❍ ❍ ❍ ❍

10. Y.W.'s mother has just arrived in the United States and speaks no English. What measures can be taken to facilitate communication between medical personnel and the mother? ❍ ❍ ❍ ❍ ❍

11. Y.W.'s mother will need a place to stay while in the United States. What can you do to facilitate the initial contact with the Thai community? ❍ ❍ ❍ ❍ ❍

12. What special discharge planning considerations are there in this case? ❍ ❍ ❍ ❍ ❍

Case Study 11

Name ____________________ Class/Group ______ Date ______

Group Members ________________________________

INSTRUCTIONS: All questions apply to this case study. Your responses should be brief and to the point. Adequate space has been provided for answers. When asked to provide several answers, they should be listed in order of priority or significance. Do not assume information that is not provided. Please print or write clearly. If your response is not legible, it will be marked as ? and you will need to rewrite it.

Scenario

G.B.'s family reports that he has had progressive back pain since his decompression laminectomy 4 months ago and is now unable to walk. He has become increasingly confused over the past 2 weeks, has occasional SOB, and is now unable to care for himself. He looks dehydrated and possibly septic. G.B. is very angry at being brought to the hospital and states, "I had this back worked on 4 months ago and I don't intend to have it done again!" G.B. is 72 years old and has had multiple health problems including GI hemorrhages, hypertension (HTN), elevated glucose, chronic lymphocytic leukemia (CLL), a remote history of kidney stones, an appendectomy, shrapnel from WW II, and a fracture (fx) of the R femur from a mining accident. His family reports that G.B. was allergic to penicillin as a child but cannot remember what reaction he experienced.

1. Based on the previous information, review the following list of admission orders. Place an "I" by each inappropriate order and state why it is inappropriate.

___ Routine VS

___ Routine neuro checks

___ Up ad lib

___ Hemogram with diff, basic metabolic panel, urinalysis, ABG, PT/INR and PTT

___ O_2 to keep SaO_2 greater than 90%

___ IV $D_5\frac{1}{2}NS$ with 20 mEq of KCl/L at 100 ml/h

___ NPO

___ Cefazolin (Kefzol) 1 g IV q8h

___ Ranitidine (Zantac) 50 mg IV q8h

___ Codeine 30 mg IM q4–6h prn for pain

___ Droperidol (Inapsine) 0.25 ml IV q8h prn for nausea

___ Acetaminophen (Tylenol) 650 mg PO q4–6h prn for fever

2. Admission VS are 165/85, 76, 20, 36.7° C. Do any of the VS concern you? Explain.

3. You get the following lab results: Na 132 mmol/L, K 3.7 mmol/L, Cl 98 mmol/L, CO_2 27 mmol/L, BUN 13 mg/dL, creatinine 0.6 mg/dL, glucose 138 mg/dL, WBC 36 thou/cmm, Hgb 10.8 g/dL, Hct 31.3%, platelets 130 thou/cmm. You call the physician to report them. What orders do you anticipate in regard to a change in IV solution?

4. What part of G.B.'s PMH is consistent with the hemogram results?

5. What noninvasive diagnostic test might be done to determine G.B.'s problem?

6. Why would an MRI be contraindicated in G.B.'s case?

7. G.B.'s family had to leave the hospital for a short time. When you enter his room, you find him trying to climb over the siderails. What should you consider before applying a vest (Posey) or wrist restraints?

8. As the afternoon progresses, G.B.'s oxygen saturation decreases from 92% on 2 L O_2/nc to 82%. The physician orders oxygen by mask at 6 L. Name at least three nursing interventions that can help improve his oxygenation status?

9. Diagnostic tests reveal that G.B. has an epidural abscess near his laminectomy incision, and he is scheduled for surgery. G.B. has already stated he does not plan to have any more surgery. Do you feel he is competent to make the decision? How would you proceed with obtaining consent?

The family tells the surgeon to go ahead with the surgery, against G.B.'s wishes. It was decided that he is not competent to make the decision for himself at this time.

10. What are considerations for discharge planning?

Case Study 12

Name ______________________ Class/Group ______ Date ______

Group Members ____

INSTRUCTIONS: All questions apply to this case study. Your responses should be brief and to the point. Adequate space has been provided for answers. When asked to provide several answers, they should be listed in order of priority or significance. Do not assume information that is not provided. Please print or write clearly. If your response is not legible, it will be marked as ? and you will need to rewrite it.

Scenario

D.H., a 54-year-old resort owner, has multiple chronic medical problems including type 2 DM for 25 years, which has progressed to type 1 DM for the past 10 years; a renal transplant 5 years ago with no signs of rejection at last biopsy; HTN; and remote peptic ulcer disease (PUD). His medications include insulin, immunosuppressives, and two antihypertensives. He visited his local physician with c/o L ear, mastoid, and sinus pain. He was diagnosed with sinusitis and *Candida albicans* (thrush); cephalexin and nystatin were prescribed. Later that evening he developed N/V, hematemesis, and weakness, and he was taken to the ED. He was admitted and started on IV antibiotics, but his condition worsened throughout the night; his dyspnea increased and he developed difficulty speaking. He was flown to your tertiary referral center and was intubated en route. On arrival, D.H. had decreased LOC with periods of total unresponsiveness, weakness, and cranial nerve deficits. His diagnosis is meningitis complicated by an aspiration pneumonia and atrial fibrillation. D.H. has continued fevers and leukocytosis despite aggressive antibiotic therapy.

1. Why is D.H. at particular risk for infection?

2. Describe bacterial meningitis.

3. What is the probable route of entry of bacteria into D.H.'s brain?

4. How do you think D.H. might have developed an aspiration pneumonia?

5. What factors influenced the physicians' decision to transport D.H. from a smaller hospital to a tertiary referral center?

6. Name four tests that could be used in the diagnosis of meningitis.

7. The following is a list of D.H's medications. Indicate why he is receiving each medication.

NPH and sliding-scale regular insulin SQ

Sucralfate (Carafate) 1 g per NGT q6h

Azathioprine 100 mg in 100 ml D_5W IVPB qd

Imipenem/cilastatin sodium (Primaxin) 500 mg IVPB based on renal lab values and peak and trough values

Methylprednisolone (Solu-Medrol) 125 mg IV q8h

Digoxin 0.125 IV qd

Metronidazole (Flagyl) 500 mg IV q6h

8. The lab just called you with a glucose result of 350 mg/dl. Identify three factors that could contribute to D.H.'s elevated glucose level.

9. List seven nursing interventions for management of D.H.'s current problems.

10. List six nursing interventions to prevent complications.

11. D.H.'s family is staying at a nearby motel. His adult son brings his mother to the hospital. Mrs. H. says she just wants to stay with her husband around the clock. She states, "I took care of him for 35 years now, and I'm not going to abandon him now when he needs me the most." How would you respond?

Note: These are stressful times for all of the individuals involved. Anything nurses can do to help alleviate the stress contributes to the well-being of patients and families. In these situations, you might consider asking if the family would like to talk with a spiritual counselor.

D.H.'s infection destroyed his cadaver kidney. He developed multiple system organ failure (MSOF) and died 7 weeks later.

Case Study 13

Name ____________________ Class/Group ______ Date ______

Group Members ________________________________

INSTRUCTIONS: All questions apply to this case study. Your responses should be brief and to the point. Adequate space has been provided for answers. When asked to provide several answers, they should be listed in order of priority or significance. Do not assume information that is not provided. Please print or write clearly. If your response is not legible, it will be marked as ? and you will need to rewrite it.

Scenario

T.S. is a 76-year-old widower being seen in your outpatient clinic for a medication refill for his Parkinson's disease. He is a retired railroad engineer who derives great pleasure from collecting railroad memorabilia and taking daily walks with his dog around his neighborhood. T.S. was diagnosed with moderate (stage III) Parkinson's disease 2 years ago. He does not smoke cigarettes or drink alcohol. His PMH includes a femur fx at age 22, a cholecystectomy at age 47, and a transurethral resection of the prostate (TURP) at age 72.

1. Because of the interference of normal muscle tone and control of smooth muscle, patients with Parkinson's disease exhibit a classic triad of symptoms. Name them.

2. Parkinson's is primarily a disease affecting older adults with symptoms usually first noted in 60- to 70-year-olds. List two reasons why we are seeing a growing number of people with Parkinson's disease.

3. Symptoms vary and are highly individualized. List eight symptoms associated with Parkinson's.

Medical management of the patient with Parkinson's is usually directed toward control of symptoms with drug therapy, supportive therapy, physiotherapy, and possibly psychotherapy. Pharmacotherapy can be fairly complex in these patients because there are several types of antiparkinsonian drugs with different mechanisms of action. The physician works with the patient to achieve the most effective regimen and often involves trial-and-error periods.

4. Why can't we just give oral dopamine as replacement therapy? What medication do we give instead?

5. Levodopa is always given in combination with carbidopa. Why?

6. What are five nursing interventions to decrease the number or severity of side effects of antiparkinsonian medications?

7. What advice will the RD give T.S. about his diet?

8. T.S. asks you to explain "Parkinsonian crisis." Describe it in a way he can understand, and describe what someone should do if it occurs.

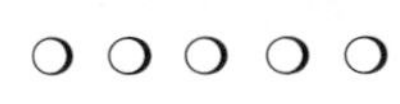

9. If you were a home health nurse, list six things that you would assess to determine whether T.S.'s care can be managed in his home. ❍ ❍ ❍ ❍ ❍

10. How might T.S's PMH affect his symptoms? ❍ ❍ ❍ ❍ ❍

For additional information, contact:
Parkinson's Disease Foundation, Inc.
710 West 168th St.
New York, NY 10032-9982
Telephone (800) 457-6676
Website: *http://www.pdf.org*

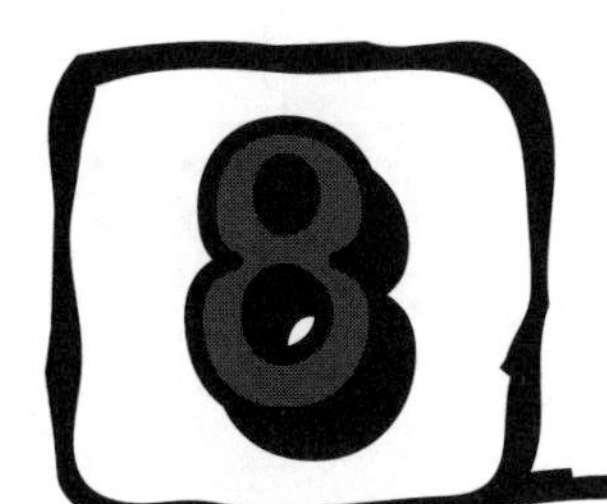

Endocrine Disorders

Case Study 1

Name ____________________ Class/Group ______ Date ______

Group Members ________________________________

INSTRUCTIONS: All questions apply to this case study. Your responses should be brief and to the point. Adequate space has been provided for answers. When asked to provide several answers, they should be listed in order of priority or significance. Do not assume information that is not provided. Please print or write clearly. If your response is not legible, it will be marked as ? and you will need to rewrite it.

❍ ❍ ❍ / ❍ ❍

Scenario

You are volunteering at a Health Fair being conducted at a local community health clinic in a large metropolitan area. You are assigned to work with an advanced practice nurse in diabetes management and are assisting in the screening process for hyperglycemia and high WHR (waist-hip ratio). During the course of the day you meet M.M., a 42-year-old African-American woman, who you suspect has some type of diabetes mellitus. A nursing history reveals the following findings: Ht 5'6", Wt 210 lb, WHR = 1.12. Her VS are 192/146, 88, 18, 98.6° F. M.M.'s mother, age 72, and two maternal aunts have type 2 diabetes mellitus (DM). M.M. has smoked 1½ packs/day of cigarettes for over 25 years and admits she should get more exercise. Screening glucose level (finger stick) is 310 mg/dL. On interview, M.M.'s only complaint is increasing fatigue over the past month and mild nocturia.

Note: Use the following reference (or the most recent version) to answer diagnostic and standards questions in this case and all diabetes cases in this chapter: Expert committee on the diagnosis and classification of diabetes mellitus, *Diabetes Care* 20:1183, 1997.

1. List the major risk factors for type 2 DM. Place a check mark next to the risk factors that M.M. has. ❍ ❍ ❍ ❍ ❍

2. What manifestation of type 2 DM is present in M.M.'s nursing history findings? ❍ ❍ ❍ ❍ ❍

3. Differentiate between a screening (or casual) plasma glucose, a fasting plasma glucose (FPG), a 2-hour postload glucose (2hPG), and HgA1c. Identify the data used to arrive at a definitive diagnosis.

   Note: The oral glucose tolerance test is rarely used in practice anymore.

4. During a brief physical assessment, the practitioner checks M.M.'s eyes with an ophthalmoscope. Why?

5. M.M. tells you she has a neighbor who had to start taking insulin for diabetes after she had "bad pneumonia." Her neighbor is very thin. M.M. asks whether she will need insulin and whether she will lose weight like her neighbor. How would you respond to her (in plain English)?

6. M.M. tells you that she knows if she would just stop eating "sweet things" she would not have diabetes. How would you correct her understanding of the disease using understandable terminology?

7. During the interview, the nurse takes M.M.'s BP and asks whether she's ever been told she has heart trouble (CAD). Explain why.

8. Discuss two modifiable behaviors M.M. engages in that will aggravate the pathologic effects of her type 2 DM.

9. In order of significance, what health problems r/t type 2 DM should be addressed?

10. M.M. agreed to come to the clinic for help; her HbA1c was 13%. What does this tell you about M.M.'s glucose control in the past few months?

11. Identify three content areas of diabetes education that are important for patients with newly diagnosed diabetes. Identify three important learning objectives for each content area.

12. Discuss two recommendations you would make to individuals participating in the Health Fair regarding primary prevention of diabetes.

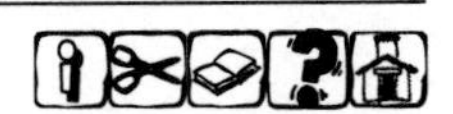

13. Explain why blood glucose testing is recommended to monitor glucose rather than urine dipstick testing. ❍ ❍ ❍ ❍ ❍

For further information, consult the American Diabetes Association Web site:
http://www.diabetes.org

Case Study 2

Name ______________________ Class/Group ______ Date ______

Group Members ____

INSTRUCTIONS: All questions apply to this case study. Your responses should be brief and to the point. Adequate space has been provided for answers. When asked to provide several answers, they should be listed in order of priority or significance. Do not assume information that is not provided. Please print or write clearly. If your response is not legible, it will be marked as ? and you will need to rewrite it.

Scenario

You graduated 3 months ago and are working with a home care nursing agency. Included in your caseload is J.S., a 60-year-old man suffering from chronic obstructive pulmonary disease (COPD). He has been on home oxygen, 2 L O_2/nc, for several years. Approximately 2 months ago, he was started on steroid therapy. Medications include metaproterenol (Alupent) inhaler, theophylline (Theo-Dur), terbutaline, dexamethasone, digoxin, and furosemide (Lasix). Not surprisingly, he also has a 50-pack-year history of cigarette smoking. On the way to visit J.S., you remember he has been progressively exhibiting s/s of Cushing's syndrome. You suspect J.S occasionally forgets to take his medication because he always seems to have "extra" pills in the bottle at the end of the month.

1. After you meet J.S., you begin an assessment and note the following findings. Place a check mark in the blank next to the s/s that characterize Cushing's syndrome.

___ Barrel chest

___ Full-looking face ("moon facies")

___ BP 180/94

___ Pursed-lip breathing, especially when patient is stressed

___ Thin arms and legs

___ Bruising on both arms

___ Acne

___ Diminished breath sounds

___ Truncal obesity with fat around clavicles and the neck

___ Weakness and fatigue

___ Impaired glucose tolerance

2. Differentiate between the cause of Cushing's syndrome and Cushing's disease.

3. Identify three to four general topics to be included in a teaching plan for J.S.

4. Identify possible consequences of suddenly stopping the dexamethasone therapy.

5. The home care nurse informs the physician of the patient's s/s. The physician decides to change J.S.'s prescription to prednisone given on alternate days. Explain the rationale for this change.

6. It is easy to forget what medications have been taken when—especially when there are several different drugs and times involved. List at least three ways you can help J.S. remember to take his pills as prescribed.

7. J.S. states that his appetite has increased but he is unable to satisfy his appetite because of SOB and he has been losing weight. How would you address this problem? How might his diet be modified?

8. You advise J.S. to take his prednisone in the morning with food and then ask him a series of questions r/t his vision. Discuss the rationale behind these nursing care actions.

9. Differentiate between the glucocorticoid and mineralocorticoid effects of prednisone.

10. How would your assessment change if J.S. were taking a glucocorticoid that also has significant mineralocorticoid activity?

11. Review J.S.'s list of medications. Based on what you know about the side effects of loop diuretics and steroids, discuss the potential problem of administering these in combination with digoxin.

12. Realizing that patients like J.S. are susceptible to all types of infections, you write guidelines to prevent infections. Identify four major points that these guidelines will include.

Case Study 3

Name ______________________ Class/Group ______ Date ______

Group Members ____

INSTRUCTIONS: All questions apply to this case study. Your responses should be brief and to the point. Adequate space has been provided for answers. When asked to provide several answers, they should be listed in order of priority or significance. Do not assume information that is not provided. Please print or write clearly. If your response is not legible, it will be marked as ? and you will need to rewrite it.

❍ ❍ ❍ / ❍ ❍

Scenario

E.H. is a 60-year-old woman who has rheumatoid arthritis. For the past 12 years, she has been taking prednisone 40 mg daily, and NSAIDs to control her disease and symptoms. As a result of her autoimmune disorder and/or long-term steroid use, E.H. has adrenal insufficiency and osteoporosis. The physician adjusts her steroid dosage for replacement therapy. In your nursing role, you are asked to conduct educational sessions designed to teach E.H. about her condition and the treatment she needs.

1. E.H. states she doesn't understand how her taking steroids has caused her body to lose its ability to produce the "the real thing." How would you explain this paradox in terms she can understand? ❍ ❍ ❍ ❍ ❍

2. People receiving steroid replacement should be taught s/s that signal the dosage is too low. What are the s/s of inadequate steroid replacement? ❍ ❍ ❍ ❍ ❍

3. What would the RD teach someone like E.H. about the nutritional implications of adrenal insufficiency? ❍ ❍ ❍ ❍ ❍

4. E.H. confides in you that she is afraid of taking steroids any longer because she has read about the deleterious effects of steroid abuse by athletes. How would you counter this misconception and alleviate E.H.'s concern?

5. How would teaching differ for this patient (on replacement therapy) as compared with teaching required for the patient taking therapeutic doses of glucocorticoids?

6. The patient states she is under a lot of stress because of her son's recent diagnosis of cancer and her husband's upcoming retirement. What are the teaching implications of this information?

7. You realize that taking exogenous cortisol can result in a variety of pathophysiologic alterations often described as Cushing's syndrome. Since E.H. will be taking lifelong steroids, would you expect to see the s/s associated with Cushing's syndrome in this individual? Explain your answer.

8. What s/s should you teach E.H. to monitor that would indicate excessive drug therapy?

9. You instruct E.H. on administration of a parenteral form of hydrocortisone. Under what circumstances should she take the parenteral form of the drug?

10. What measures should E.H. take to prevent an acute episode of adrenal insufficiency?

11. E.H. tells you she never used to take pills at all. She says she hates to be "addicted to a drug." What will you tell her?

Case Study 4

Name ____________________ Class/Group ______ Date ______

Group Members ________________________________

INSTRUCTIONS: All questions apply to this case study. Your responses should be brief and to the point. Adequate space has been provided for answers. When asked to provide several answers, they should be listed in order of priority or significance. Do not assume information that is not provided. Please print or write clearly. If your response is not legible, it will be marked as ? and you will need to rewrite it.

❍ ❍ ❍ / ❍ ❍

Scenario

You are working in a community outpatient clinic where you perform the intake assessment on R.M., a 38-year-old woman who is attending graduate school. Her CC is overwhelming fatigue that is not relieved by rest. She is so exhausted that she has difficulty walking to classes and studying. She has coarse, sparse scalp hair; scaly skin; slightly slurred speech; thick tongue; a hoarse voice; puffiness around the eyes; yellowish-colored skin and nails; and swollen neck. Initial VS were 92/64, 56, 12, 96.8° F.

1. Compare her VS with those of a healthy person her same age. ❍ ❍ ❍ ❍ ❍

2. List eight general questions you might ask R.M. to get a "ball park" idea of what is going on with her. ❍ ❍ ❍ ❍ ❍

3. You know that some of R.M.'s symptoms could be caused by depression, hypothyroidism, anemia, cardiac disease, fluid and electrolyte imbalance, or allergies. As part of your screening procedures, how would you begin to investigate which of these conditions probably do not account for R.M.'s symptoms? ❍ ❍ ❍ ❍ ❍

You find no obvious irregularities in R.M.'s cardiopulmonary assessment.

4. Unnecessary diagnostic tests are expensive. What tests do you think would be the most important for R.M., and why?

R.M.'s TSH comes back 10.9; the family nurse practitioner diagnoses R.M. with hypothyroidism and places her on thyroid replacement therapy.

5. The practitioner prescribes levothyroxine (Synthroid) 1.7 g/kg body weight/day. R.M. weighs 130 lb. What should be her daily dose of Synthroid in milligrams? How would her prescription read?

6. R.M.'s TSH level is increased. Explain the relationship between these lab results and hypothyroidism.

7. What patient teaching needs will you review with R.M. before she leaves? Remember medication issues.

8. Why would you want to obtain a complete drug history on R.M.?

9. What general teaching issues would you address with R.M.? ❍ ❍ ❍ ❍ ❍

10. R.M. wonders whether she should take iodine supplements if she decreases her salt intake. She recognizes that salt is a significant source of iodine in her part of the country. What would you explain to her? ❍ ❍ ❍ ❍ ❍

11. What should you teach R.M. regarding prevention of myxedema coma? ❍ ❍ ❍ ❍ ❍

12. Before R.M. leaves the clinic, she asks how she will know whether the medication is "doing its job." Outline simple expected outcomes for R.M. ❍ ❍ ❍ ❍ ❍

13. Several weeks later, R.M. calls the clinic stating she can't remember whether she took her thyroid medication. What additional data should you obtain, and how would you advise her?

14. Under what circumstances should R.M. hold the drug or call the clinic?

R.M. comes in 2 months later for a follow-up visit. You can't believe she is the same person. She looks and walks as if she were 10 years younger. Her skin appears more moist, and her hair is beginning to come in with its normal feel. "You can't believe how much different I'm feeling," she says. "I'm discovering what it's like to live again."

Case Study 5

Name ______________________ Class/Group ______ Date ______

Group Members ______________________________

INSTRUCTIONS: All questions apply to this case study. Your responses should be brief and to the point. Adequate space has been provided for answers. When asked to provide several answers, they should be listed in order of priority or significance. Do not assume information that is not provided. Please print or write clearly. If your response is not legible, it will be marked as ? and you will need to rewrite it.

Scenario

You are working on an oncology unit and will be receiving a patient from the recovery room. The post-anesthesia care unit (PACU) nurse calls and gives the following report. C.P., a 50-year-old woman, had a total thyroidectomy (multinodular goiter), left superior and right inferior parathyroidectomy because of adenoma. The estimated blood loss (EBL) was 25 ml. VS are 130/82, 80-90, 20. She has a peripheral IV of $D_5\frac{1}{2}$NS with 20 mEq KCl and 10 mEq calcium gluconate infusing at 100 ml/h. She has received a total of 50 mg meperidine IVP, and she remains AAO. C.P.'s PMH includes total abdominal hysterectomy (TAH) for fibroids and low-level radiation treatments to the neck 38 years ago for eczema. Her medications include estradiol, lovastatin, and levothyroxine. Both parents are living; her father had an MI at 70 years old, her mother has hypothyroidism but never had thyroid tumors. Preoperative laboratory findings: Ca 11.2 mg/dl, phosphorus 2.4 mg/dl, Cl 106 mmol/L, alkaline phosphatase 112 U/L, elevated parahormone and TSH levels, creatinine 1.4 mg/dL.

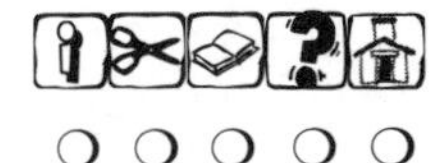

1. What additional data should you obtain from the recovery room nurse?

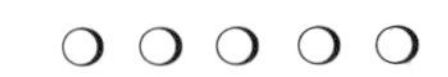

2. What preparations will you take before C.P. arrives?

3. You receive C.P. from the recovery room. How will you focus your initial assessment, and why?

4. During your initial assessment, you document negative Chvostek's and Trousseau's signs. Describe data that would support this conclusion.

5. Explain why C.P. would have been taking Synthroid preoperatively.

6. Identify the major risk factor that may have contributed to the development of parathyroid adenoma in C.P.

7. Identify four nursing issues r/t C.P.'s care.

8. Identify four nursing actions you should include in the postoperative care of C.P.

9. Identify nursing care measures that reduce the risk for postoperative swelling.

10. The next day, 24 hours after surgery, C.P. calls you into her room c/o numbness around her mouth and tingling at the tips of her fingers. She appears restless but is AAO. Realizing that C.P. may be experiencing hypocalcemia, you decide to notify the physician. What should you do in the interim before the physician returns your call?

11. What emergency equipment should you gather?

C.P. is given supplemental calcium gluconate and recovers without further complications. C.P. is being discharged 48 hours postoperatively. She states that she can't wait until she can stop taking the Synthroid.

12. How would you respond to her statement?

Case Study 6

Name ______________________ Class/Group ______ Date ______

Group Members ____

INSTRUCTIONS: All questions apply to this case study. Your responses should be brief and to the point. Adequate space has been provided for answers. When asked to provide several answers, they should be listed in order of priority or significance. Do not assume information that is not provided. Please print or write clearly. If your response is not legible, it will be marked as ? and you will need to rewrite it.

Scenario

K.B. is an 80-year-old woman admitted to the hospital following a 5-day episode of the "flu" with c/o DOE (dyspnea on exertion), palpitations, chest pain, insomnia, and fatigue. Her PMH includes congestive heart failure (CHF) and hypertension (HTN) requiring antihypertensive medications (she states that she has not been taking these medications on a regular basis). K.B. was diagnosed with Graves' disease 6 months ago and was placed on propylthiouracil (PTU) 100 mg PO q6h. Assessment findings are as follows: Ht 5'2", Wt 100 lb. Appears anxious and restless. Loud heart sounds. VS are 150/90, 104 irregular, 20, 100.2° F; 1+ pitting edema noted in lower extremities. Diminished breath sounds with fine crackles in the posterior bases. K.B. states she recently lost her husband. Laboratory findings: Hgb 11.8 g/dL, Hct 36%, erythrocyte sedimentation rate (ESR) 48 mm/h, Na 141 mmol/L, K 4.7 mmol/L, Cl 101 mmol/L, BUN 33 mg/dL, creatinine 1.9 mg/dL, T_4 14.0 g/dL, T_3 230 mg/dL.

1. Of the physical assessment and laboratory findings, which represent manifestations of hypermetabolism?

2. What additional subjective and objective data would you gather for someone with Graves' disease?

3. After AM rounds, the physician leaves the following orders. Which of the orders would you question and why?
   Propranolol (Inderal) 20 mg PO q6h
   Dexamethasone (Decadron) 10 mg IV q6h
   Verapamil (Calan SR) 120 mg PO qd
   Diet as tolerated, high-protein
   STAT ECG
   Up ad lib

4. Develop four priority nursing problems r/t K.B.'s care.

5. Later on your shift, you note that K.B. is extremely restless and is disoriented to person, place, and time. VS are 104/62, 180 and irregular, 32 and labored, 104° F. Her ECG shows atrial fibrillation. What do these findings indicate?

6. What would you do first?

K.B. is in thyroid crisis. The physician orders the following: STAT ABGs; digoxin (Lanoxin) 0.125 mg IVP q8h x 3 doses; IV of D_5W at 100 ml/h; Lugol's solution (strong iodine) 10 drops PO tid; increase propylthiouracil (PTU) to 200 mg PO qid; hydrocortisone (Hydro-Cort) 100 mg IVP q8h; cardiac monitor; absolute bed rest; cooling blanket for temp >102° F; acetaminophen (Tylenol) 650 mg PO prn temp >100° F.

7. Why did the physician order acetaminophen instead of salicylates?

8. Identify four nursing measures that would be essential in caring for K.B.

9. Identify two possible contributing factors that may have precipitated K.B.'s thyroid storm.

10. Before discharge, the physician discusses 2 treatment options with K.B. and her family: radioactive iodine (RAI) therapy using ^{131}I, and subtotal thyroidectomy. K.B. is fearful of radiation treatment and asks you for your opinion. How would you respond?

11. K.B. decides to receive ^{131}I. During pretreatment instructions, the family asks if she will be radioactive and what precautions they should take. Outline important guidelines for instructing K.B. and her family on home precautions.

12. Discuss how your discharge teaching instructions will differ from those you would give to someone following a subtotal thyroidectomy.

❍ ❍ ❍ ❍ ❍

Case Study 8

Name ______________________ Class/Group ______ Date ______

Group Members ______________________________

INSTRUCTIONS: All questions apply to this case study. Your responses should be brief and to the point. Adequate space has been provided for answers. When asked to provide several answers, they should be listed in order of priority or significance. Do not assume information that is not provided. Please print or write clearly. If your response is not legible, it will be marked as ? and you will need to rewrite it.

❍ ❍ ❍ / ❍ ❍

Scenario

W.V., a 40-year-old woman, has been referred to the endocrine clinic of a large metropolitan medical center by her primary care physician. She presents with a history of bilateral hemianopsia, headaches, menstrual disturbances (amenorrhea), dyspareunia, and lethargy. An extensive history reveals polyuria and polydipsia. Her family physician suspects an anterior pituitary tumor. GH, prolactin, TSH, LH, and FSH levels are unremarkable. A dexamethasone suppression test (or cortisol/ACTH challenge test) and 24-hour urine for 17-hydroxysteroids (17-OHCS) are planned.

1. W.V. is aware of the high probability of a pituitary tumor, but she doesn't understand why the physician wants to test her kidneys. How would you explain the relationship between the pituitary and adrenal glands and the need for adrenal function studies to her? ❍ ❍ ❍ ❍ ❍

2. Identify four nursing problems r/t W.V.'s care. ❍ ❍ ❍ ❍ ❍

The dexamethasone suppression test is normal, but the 24-hour urine for 17-OHCS is elevated. An MRI is ordered.

3. The MRI confirms a macroadenoma of the anterior pituitary. The physician advises a transsphenoidal hypophysectomy. What questions would you anticipate W.V. might have?

4. While W.V.'s physician arranges for her admission to the hospital and schedules her transsphenoidal hypophysectomy, you enter her examining room to conduct preop teaching. You find W.V. crying. She says she is embarrassed by the hormonal changes and states, "I'm afraid my husband won't love me anymore." What approaches would be appropriate for addressing the patient's fear?

5. During preop teaching, W.V. states she is fearful of the procedure. She says she doesn't understand how a tumor in the brain can be removed through the nose. How would you explain the procedure to minimize her fear?

6. Identify two major teaching needs for postop care based on the transsphenoidal approach. Outline important educational points for each area to address during preop teaching with W.V.

7. W.V. is admitted and undergoes a successful transsphenoidal hypophysectomy. Ten hours postop, W.V. calls her nurse into her room c/o postnasal drip. She is frequently swallowing. What five actions should the nurse take? Include your rationales.

8. The nurse notes the following assessment findings: VS 100/66, 98, 16; W.V. c/o thirst; her skin is flushed; her urine output 300 ml/h with a specific gravity of 1.003, and she is flaccid (e.g., no muscle tone). What additional information should you gather before calling the physician?

9. The nurse suspects fluid volume deficit r/t inadequate release of ADH. While waiting for the surgeon to return her call, what should the nurse's priority intervention(s) be?

10. The surgeon orders a serum and urine osmolality and electrolytes. The lab reports a urine osmolality of 95 mOsm/kg, serum osmolality of 315 mOsm/kg, and sodium level of 146 mmol/L. Discuss the significance of each.

11. Replacement therapy for diabetes insipidus includes administration of aqueous vasopressin (Pitressin) or the synthetic vasopressin analog desmopressin (DDAVP). Compare the advantage(s) and disadvantage(s) of using desmopressin versus aqueous Pitressin in this situation.

12. How will the nurse evaluate the effectiveness of drug and fluid therapy?

Case Study 9

Name ______________________ Class/Group ______ Date ______

Group Members ____

INSTRUCTIONS: All questions apply to this case study. Your responses should be brief and to the point. Adequate space has been provided for answers. When asked to provide several answers, they should be listed in order of priority or significance. Do not assume information that is not provided. Please print or write clearly. If your response is not legible, it will be marked as ? and you will need to rewrite it.

Scenario

You are a nurse on a medical unit. One of your patients, T.L., a 40-year-old man who works as a communications supervisor, is being evaluated for uncontrolled HTN. He c/o frequent episodes of chest pain and palpitations, diaphoresis, job stress, nervousness, epigastric distress after eating, and pounding migraine headaches that leave him exhausted. He states that these episodes have increased in frequency and duration; he now experiences several episodes a week, and each episode lasts 1 to 3 days. He has taken a variety of antihypertensive medications, none of which have successfully controlled his HTN. His BP is labile; sometimes it is normal, and other times it is 220/120. Cardiac workup reveals no significant cardiovascular abnormalities. He has a 27-pack-year smoking history. T.L.'s 24-hour urine analysis reveals: vanillylmandelic acid (VMA) 12 mg/24h; epinephrine 45 ng/24h, and norepinephrine 100 ng/24h; CT scan reveals a single adrenomedullary tumor. T.L. is diagnosed with pheochromocytoma and scheduled for an adrenalectomy.

1. The physician informs T.L. that an adrenal tumor is causing his symptoms. T.L. is obviously upset with his diagnosis. He states he doesn't understand how a tumor on top of his kidney can cause high BP. He asks whether this means he has cancer. How would you respond?

2. The physician advises T.L. to undergo an adrenalectomy. He is immediately started on phenoxybenzamine (Dibenzyline) 20 mg PO q8h, and propranolol (Inderal) 40 mg PO bid. What is the connection between these two drugs and the diagnosis?

3. Some people experience paroxysmal, or sudden, periodic attacks of HTN that correspond to the release of epinephrine and/or norepinephrine. Under what circumstances would T.L. most likely experience a paroxysmal hypertensive event?

4. What measures to prevent a paroxysmal hypertensive event should you teach T.L.?

5. T.L. is given hydrocortisone (Solu-Cortef) 100 mg IV push preoperatively. Discuss the significance of this drug in the preoperative period.

6. Following the surgery, T.L. is taken directly to the ICU. The anesthesiologist gives the admitting nurse the following report: the surgery went well, and T.L. should wake up shortly; his VS have been running 180/90, 88, 16, 96.1° F; he's got a left subclavian Swan-Ganz catheter and 2 large-bore peripheral IVs with D_5W running at a total of 125 ml/h; urine output during OR was 200 ml. What additional data should the ICU nurse elicit from the anesthesiologist?

7. Identify three postoperative nursing issues r/t T.L.'s care.

8. For each nursing care issue identified in question 7, outline two to three nursing interventions/measures.

9. During shift assessment (second postop day), the nurse notes that T.L. seems less alert, his grip strength is markedly weaker than yesterday, and his mucous membranes are dry. The previous nurse reported that he had vomited twice in the last hour. The cardiac monitor shows peaked T waves and a widened QRS complex. VS are 120/72, 94, 14, 101° F. What conclusions can you draw from the above data?

All of these findings suggest adrenal insufficiency.

10. Based on the nurses' assessment findings, what general treatment measures would you anticipate?

11. Outline four nursing care measures that are critical during this period.

12. T.L. is stabilized and is scheduled to be discharged to home. During discharge teaching, T.L. asks whether he will require steroids for the rest of his life. How should you respond to T.L.?

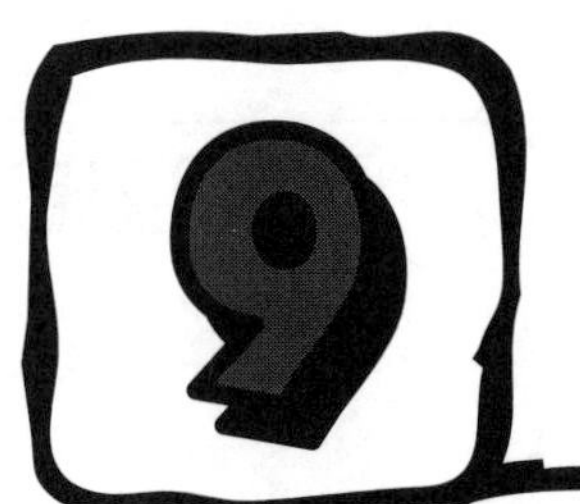

Immunologic Disorders

Case Study 1

Name ______________________ Class/Group ______ Date ______

Group Members ____________________________________

INSTRUCTIONS: All questions apply to this case study. Your responses should be brief and to the point. Adequate space has been provided for answers. When asked to provide several answers, they should be listed in order of priority or significance. Do not assume information that is not provided. Please print or write clearly. If your response is not legible, it will be marked as ? and you will need to rewrite it.

Scenario

You are a nurse at the student health center (SHC) at a local university. T.Q., a 19-year-old male student, visits the clinic on the first day of autumn quarter to inform you of his immunodeficiency problem. He gives you a letter from his attending physician, a vial of gamma globulin, and asks you to give him his "shot." The letter, written by T.Q.'s physician, states that he was diagnosed with primary immunodeficiency disease 4 years ago. He has an adequate number of B-cells but inadequate numbers of immunoglobulin. T.Q. has a history of chronic sinus and upper respiratory tract infections and occasional GI tract infections. He is maintained on 0.66 ml/kg gamma globulin IV every 3 weeks. T.Q. responds well to his treatment and has suffered no side effects from gamma globulin other than occasional redness at the injection site. T.Q. has no other known illnesses or allergies and is on tetracycline for acne. T.Q. is 5'11", weighs 190 lb, and has several pustular lesions on his face and neck. His VS are 134/78, 84, 20, 98.8° F.

1. What actions will you take first?

2. What should you do while the physician is verifying information?

3. Would you give T.Q. his own medication?

4. What other assessments should you make before T.Q. leaves?

5. You note on T.Q.'s health record that he has not received his polio, measles, mumps, or rubella vaccines. What explanation can be given for the lack of these vaccinations?

T.Q. is very knowledgeable about his condition. After receiving his injection, he makes an appointment to return to the SHC in 3 weeks. He returns at that time with c/o a stuffy nose.

6. How should you respond to T.Q.'s complaints?

7. If T.Q. is developing a sinus infection, what signs are you likely to encounter upon examining him?

T.Q.'s nares do not appear swollen or red, although he does have some clear mucus drainage. His temperature is normal at 98.4° F. T.Q. is due for his next injection of gamma globulin.

8. Should you give the medication or ask him to return when he is no longer having nasal stuffiness? Why or why not?

9. Should any adjustments be made in T.Q.'s class schedule or activities because of his condition?

10. How do primary immunodeficiencies differ from secondary immunodeficiencies?

11. Explain why T.Q. is at greater risk for the development of infections than his classmates.

12. How do injections of gamma globulin help T.Q. fight off infections?

13. What are the major side effects that can occur from injections of gamma globulin?

14. Given the nature of side effects associated with gamma globulin, how long should T.Q. wait at the health center before leaving?

Case Study 2

Name ______________________ Class/Group ______ Date ______

Group Members ______________________________________

INSTRUCTIONS: All questions apply to this case study. Your responses should be brief and to the point. Adequate space has been provided for answers. When asked to provide several answers, they should be listed in order of priority or significance. Do not assume information that is not provided. Please print or write clearly. If your response is not legible, it will be marked as ? and you will need to rewrite it.

Scenario

You are working at a physician's office, and you have just taken C.Q., a 38-year-old woman, into the consultation room. C.Q. has been divorced for 5 years, has 2 daughters (ages 14 and 16), and works full-time as a legal secretary. Two weeks ago she visited her doctor for a routine physical examination and requested that an HIV (human immunodeficiency virus) test be performed. C.Q. stated that she was in a serious relationship, is contemplating marriage, and just wanted to make certain she was "okay." No abnormalities were noted during C.Q.'s physical examination and blood was drawn for routine blood chemistries, hematology studies, and an ELISA (enzyme-linked immunosorbent assay) test, also known as the EIA (enzyme immunoassay) test. C.Q. is at the office to receive her lab results. The physician informs you that C.Q.'s EIA was positive.

1. What is an EIA test? Does a positive EIA mean that C.Q. definitely has HIV?

2. You explain to C.Q. that one of her tests needs to be repeated and you need to draw another blood sample. Why wouldn't you tell C.Q. that her first test result was positive and that another test is needed before the diagnosis can be confirmed?

The physician informs you that C.Q.'s Western blot test results confirm that she is HIV-positive; he requests that you be present when he talks to her. Before leaving C.Q.'s room, the physician requests that you obtain another blood sample for further testing, give C.Q. verbal and written information about local AIDS support groups, and help C.Q. call a friend to accompany her home this evening. She looks at you through her tears and states, "I can't believe it. J. is the only man I've had sex with since my divorce. He told me I had nothing to worry about. I can't believe he would do this to me."

3. C.Q.'s statement is based on three assumptions: that J. is HIV-positive, that he intentionally withheld the information from her, and that he intentionally transmitted the HIV to her through unprotected sex. Based on your knowledge of HIV infection, how would you counsel C.Q.?

4. In addition to offering alternative explanations and exploring options, what is your most important role at this time?

5. Identify at least three nursing issues r/t to C.Q.'s care.

6. C.Q. has had a positive EIA test and is seropositive for HIV. Why doesn't she have s/s of AIDS?

7. What assessment findings would support a diagnoses of AIDS?

8. Why is it a good idea that someone C.Q. trusts escort her home this evening?

C.Q. gives you the name and phone number of a relative she wants you to call. You remain with her until she leaves with her relative.

9. Has C.Q.'s right to privacy been violated? Explain why or why not?

10. C.Q. returns to the office 4 days later to discuss her diagnosis. What issues will you discuss with her at this time?

11. Does C.Q. have a legal responsibility to inform J. of her HIV status?

Two weeks later C.Q. visits the office and asks to speak to you in private. She thanks you for talking to her the day she received the news of her diagnosis. She pulls a gun from her purse and states, "I was going to go out into the waiting room and blow J. away, because I thought he was cheating on me." She tells you that J. confessed to her he was afraid to tell her about his hemophilia because she might leave him. J. is tested for HIV at regular intervals and his last HIV test, 6 months ago, had been negative. J. was retested, and this test was positive for HIV. J.'s doctor discussed the possibility of transmission through recombinant factor VIII products. C.Q. tells you that they are going to get married and invites you to the wedding. She stops at the door and says, "At least we won't have to worry about 'safe sex' with each other!"

Case Study 3

Name ______________________ Class/Group ______ Date ______

Group Members ____

INSTRUCTIONS: All questions apply to this case study. Your responses should be brief and to the point. Adequate space has been provided for answers. When asked to provide several answers, they should be listed in order of priority or significance. Do not assume information that is not provided. Please print or write clearly. If your response is not legible, it will be marked as ? and you will need to rewrite it.

❍ ❍ ❍ / ❍ ❍

Scenario

J.P., a 56-year-old man, developed a severe viral infection and suffered fatigue, fever, and myalgia. Although he recovered from the acute episode, J.P. never quite regained normal activity level. Six months later, J.P. continues to find it difficult to work a 10-hour day as a brick mason so he returns to his physician. Diagnostic studies reveal CHF r/t postviral cardiomyopathy. Following medical management with digoxin (Lanoxin) and furosemide (Lasix), his condition stabilizes and he returns to work, but his attendance is erratic. J.P.'s condition gradually deteriorates, and he is readmitted to the hospital 16 months later with c/o dyspnea with minimal exertion, fatigue, orthopnea, chest pain, anorexia, and feelings of abdominal fullness. He has 1+ peripheral edema and is diaphoretic. Further studies reveal that J.P. has cardiac dilation, moderate to gross ventricular hypertrophy, and poor systolic ejection fraction, consistent with severe congestive cardiomyopathy. Because J.P.'s only other health problem is mild hypertension, heart transplant evaluation is recommended. J.P. and his wife discuss his prognosis and agree to an evaluation for possible heart transplantation.

1. If J.P. is accepted for cardiac transplantation, what data will be collected in addition to his past medical history, current diagnostic findings, and cardiac evaluation? ❍ ❍ ❍ ❍ ❍

2. What criteria for heart transplantation does J.P. meet that will make him eligible for cardiac transplantation? ❍ ❍ ❍ ❍ ❍

3. Cite five contraindications for cardiac transplant. ❍ ❍ ❍ ❍ ❍

4. J.P. is accepted for cardiac transplant and placed on the waiting list. What fears or concerns may J.P. experience during this waiting period?

J.P. receives a phone call to report to the hospital immediately because a donor heart has become available.

5. What compatibility tests are performed to determine eligibility for transplantation and to ensure as close a match as possible?

6. As the nurse on the transplant unit, how can you best help J.P. prepare for his heart transplant?

J.P.'s surgery and recovery are uncomplicated and he is sent home and referred to cardiac rehabilitation after adjustment of his immunosuppression therapy and appropriate teaching. J.P. is readmitted for low grade fever and dyspnea 6 weeks after surgery. Cardiac biopsies demonstrate moderate acute rejection.

7. What is the etiology of acute rejection, and how does it differ from chronic rejection?

8. The nurse can anticipate that prompt immunosuppressive therapy will be instituted using what drug? How does this drug alter the rejection process? ❍ ❍ ❍ ❍ ❍

9. What is the most important nursing intervention for J.P. at this time, and why? ❍ ❍ ❍ ❍ ❍

J.P. responds positively to steroid therapy and is released to home after 5 days. J.P. is again admitted to the hospital with renewed c/o of dyspnea, low-grade fever, and ankle swelling 7 months later. Both J.P. and his wife are anxious and fearful.

10. Explain what may be happening to J.P. physiologically. ❍ ❍ ❍ ❍ ❍

11. How will treatment for this episode of graft rejection differ from treatment for his earlier episode of rejection? ❍ ❍ ❍ ❍ ❍

12. J.P.'s prognosis for the future will depend on what factors? ❍ ❍ ❍ ❍ ❍

Case Study 4

Name ______________________ Class/Group ______ Date ______

Group Members ____

INSTRUCTIONS: All questions apply to this case study. Your responses should be brief and to the point. Adequate space has been provided for answers. When asked to provide several answers, they should be listed in order of priority or significance. Do not assume information that is not provided. Please print or write clearly. If your response is not legible, it will be marked as ? and you will need to rewrite it.

❍ ❍ ❍ / ❍ ❍

Scenario

W.V. is a 47-year-old man who lives with his wife and 2 teen-age sons. W.V. developed chronic renal failure 12 years ago after acute renal failure due to phenacetin use. (W.V. took phenacetin for years since his early 20s for migraine headaches. Large doses of phenacetin over the years can cause analgesic-induced nephropathy. This drug has subsequently been removed from the market.) W.V. was initially placed on hemodialysis but was switched to peritoneal dialysis so he could remain employed as an auto mechanic. Three months ago W.V. received a cadaveric transplant, or cadaver kidney. He recovered without complications and his serum laboratory values returned to normal. He was placed on immunosuppressive therapy, including cyclosporine and prednisone and was discharged to home. W.V. returned to work 3 weeks later.

Today W.V. reports to his physician for routine follow-up. His VS are 148/92, 88, 24, 99.2° F. His lab data reveal the following: serum creatinine 1.2 mg/dL, BUN 22 mg/dL, normal serum electrolytes. W.V. has gained 5 pounds since discharge from the hospital.

1. What histocompatibility studies are generally performed before renal transplant, and why are they important? ❍ ❍ ❍ ❍ ❍

2. By what criteria is W.V. considered a good candidate for renal transplantation? ❍ ❍ ❍ ❍ ❍

3. If W.V.'s kidney is producing sufficient urine and he is feeling well, why is it necessary to monitor his laboratory data? ❍ ❍ ❍ ❍ ❍

4. What is the possible significance of W.V.'s current BP?

5. How does the drug cyclosporine protect W.V.'s kidney from rejection, and what are the most important side effects of this drug that W.V. must be taught to monitor?

6. How will W.V. know whether he is experiencing organ rejection?

7. If W.V. begins to reject his kidney, how would the rejection be classified, and what s/s would most likely be present?

8. Identify at least four ways that W.V. might experience difficulty adjusting to his organ transplant.

9. How can you best support W.V. and his family? ❍ ❍ ❍ ❍ ❍

10. Why is it necessary for W.V. to be concerned about infection? ❍ ❍ ❍ ❍ ❍

Case Study 5

Name ________________________ Class/Group ______ Date ______

Group Members ____

INSTRUCTIONS: All questions apply to this case study. Your responses should be brief and to the point. Adequate space has been provided for answers. When asked to provide several answers, they should be listed in order of priority or significance. Do not assume information that is not provided. Please print or write clearly. If your response is not legible, it will be marked as ? and you will need to rewrite it.

Scenario

K.D. is a 36-year-old gay professional man who has been HIV-positive for 6 years. Until recently, he demonstrated no s/s of AIDS. The appearance of purplish spots on his neck and arms persuaded him to make an appointment with his physician. Upon arrival at the doctor's office, the nurse performs a brief assessment. His VS are 138/86, 100, 30, 100.8° F. K.D. states that he has been feeling fatigued for several months and is experiencing occasional night sweats but he also has been working long hours, has skipped meals, and has been particularly stressed over a project at work. K.D.'s physical is WNL except for his low-grade fever and skin lesions. The doctor orders a CBC, lymphocyte studies, and a PPD. K.D. made an appointment to return in 5 days to discuss the results of his tests.

Over the next 2 weeks, K.D. develops a fever of 101° F, nonproductive cough, and increasing SOB. Late one night he becomes acutely SOB, so his roommate, J.F., takes him to the ED where he is subsequently admitted to the hospital with probable *Pneumocystis carinii* pneumonia. Bronchoalveolar lavage examined under light microscopy confirms the diagnosis. K.D.'s admission WBC and lymphocyte studies demonstrate an increased pattern of immunodeficiency from earlier studies. K.D. is placed on nasal oxygen, IV fluids, and IV trimethoprim/sulfamethoxadole.

1. What is *Pneumocystis carinii* pneumonia (PCP)?

2. What is the significance of the purplish spots over K.D.'s neck and arms?

3. Identify four nursing diagnoses for K.D.

4. What precautions will you need to use when caring for K.D.?

5. What will be the focus of your ongoing assessment? (List five.)

6. What major side effects of his antibiotic should you monitor K.D. for?

7. Differentiate between HIV-positive status and AIDS.

8. Why is K.D.'s development of PCP of particular importance in light of his HIV status?

9. K.D. has been seropositive for several years, yet he has been asymptomatic for AIDS. What factors may have influenced K.D.'s development of pneumocystis?

K.D. is responding well to treatment, and plans are being made for discharge. He will be started on standard therapy, with follow-up on an outpatient basis. Since "standard therapy" changes in response to developments in clinical research, you will have to look up the most recent recommended treatment.

10. K.D. was taught about disease transmission and safe sex, and encouraged to maintain moderate exercise, rest, and dietary habits when he was first diagnosed as HIV-positive. Give at least four additional topics that should be discussed with K.D. before he goes home.

11. What laboratory data will most likely be monitored on K.D. in the future? ❍ ❍ ❍ ❍ ❍

12. List at least five other opportunistic infections that K.D. is at risk for developing. ❍ ❍ ❍ ❍ ❍

For additional information, check the following resources.

National Institute of Allergy and Infectuous Diseases: *http://www.niaid.nih.gov/* and *http://www.niaid.nih.gov/publications/hivaids/hivaids.htm*

Another comprehensive source of information: *http://www.thebody.com/*

Case Study 6

Name ______________________ Class/Group ______ Date ______

Group Members ____

INSTRUCTIONS: All questions apply to this case study. Your responses should be brief and to the point. Adequate space has been provided for answers. When asked to provide several answers, they should be listed in order of priority or significance. Do not assume information that is not provided. Please print or write clearly. If your response is not legible, it will be marked as ? and you will need to rewrite it.

Scenario

D.C. is a 32-year-old white clerical worker who lives with his 76-year-old grandmother, his primary caregiver. He was diagnosed as being HIV-positive 3 months ago and has been under close outpatient medical supervision for the past 3 weeks because of persistent fever, pulmonary infiltrates, and nonspecific flu-like symptoms. He is admitted to your nursing unit for fever, chills, sweats, myalgias, malaise, chest pain, dry nonproductive cough, axillary adenopathy, N/V, and severe diarrhea. Admission VS are 108/84, 104, 30, 103.5° F. Following aggressive diagnostic workup, D.C. is diagnosed with AIDS complicated by *Pneumocystis carinii* pneumonia, cryptosporidiosis, oral candidiasis, and cytomegalovirus (CMV) infection.

Today is D.C.'s third day postadmission to the hospital. He remains acutely ill; however, his hydration status has improved, and he is experiencing fewer than 8 diarrhea stools per day. He is not yet able to keep food or fluids down; therefore, TPN is being considered. D.C. has c/o headache, nausea, continued fatigue, and muscle soreness. He is able to ambulate to the bathroom with assistance.

1. Why was D.C. diagnosed as having AIDS rather than complicated HIV infection?

2. Considering D.C.'s AIDS status, what findings are likely to be present when you receive the results of his lymphocyte studies?

3. Provide a possible explanation for D.C.'s rapid conversion from HIV positive to AIDS.

4. As D.C.'s nurse, list at least two observations you would monitor in relation to each of the following infections: cryptosporidiosis, candidiasis, and CMV.

5. Given the previous possible problems that D.C. could encounter, which of the following nursing orders would be appropriate? Label each with "A" for appropriate or "I" for inappropriate and correct the inappropriate orders.

___ Monitor VS q12h.

___ Assist with ADL as needed.

___ Keep perineal area clean and dry; use protective skin cream.

___ Regular diet.

___ Monitor lungs, skin, abdomen, and urine output once per shift.

___ Maintain complete bed rest.

___ Use toothettes or soft-bristled brush for oral hygiene.

___ Exclude diarrhea stool from I&O measurements.

___ Monitor IV site for signs of inflammation; change site if red or swollen.

6. D.C. is restless at times because of his muscle soreness. Upon entering his room, you note that he has pulled out his peripheral IV and is bleeding. How should you respond?

7. Cite at least five findings that would indicate D.C.'s condition is stabilizing or improving.

8. What assessment findings would the physician take into consideration when making the decision to place D.C. on TPN?

9. Given that D.C.'s grandmother is his primary caregiver, discuss the implications of D.C.'s diagnosis of AIDS.

10. Would D.C. require additional teaching regarding his ability to transmit HIV now that he has AIDS?

11. D.C. begins to slowly respond to treatment, and discharge plans are begun. Identify at least three ways that D.C.'s post-AIDS care will differ from his pre-AIDS care.

Note: Advances and changes are occurring too rapidly for specific questions. Check authoritative Internet resources for the most recent information.

Case Study 7

Name ______________________ Class/Group ______ Date ______

Group Members ____

INSTRUCTIONS: All questions apply to this case study. Your responses should be brief and to the point. Adequate space has been provided for answers. When asked to provide several answers, they should be listed in order of priority or significance. Do not assume information that is not provided. Please print or write clearly. If your response is not legible, it will be marked as ? and you will need to rewrite it.

Scenario

D.W. is a 23-year-old married woman with 3 children under the age of 5. She presented to her physician 2 years ago with vague c/o intermittent fatigue, joint pain, and low-grade fever. Her physician noted small patchy areas of vitiligo and a scaly rash across her nose, cheeks, back, and chest at that time. Laboratory studies revealed that D.W. had a positive antinuclear antibody titer, positive lupus erythematosus (LE) cell prep, elevated C-reactive protein and ESR, and decreased C_3 and C_4 serum complement. Joint x-rays demonstrated joint swelling without joint erosion. D.W. was subsequently diagnosed with systemic lupus erythematosus (SLE). She was initially treated with sulindac 200 mg PO bid and prednisone 20 mg PO qd, bed rest, ice packs, and aspirin to control discomfort. She was counseled regarding her condition, advised to balance rest and activity, eat a well-balanced diet, use strategies to reduce stress, and avoid direct sunlight. D.W. responded well to treatment and was eventually told she could report for follow-up every 6 months unless her symptoms became acute. D.W. resumed her job in environmental services at a large geriatric facility.

1. What is the significance of each of D.W.'s laboratory findings?

2. How does cutaneous lupus erythematosus differ from SLE?

3. What priority problems need to be addressed with D.W.?

Eighteen months after diagnosis, D.W. seeks out her physician because of puffy hands and feet and increased fatigue. D.W. reports that she has been working longer hours because of the absence of two of her fellow workers. Diagnostic evaluation reveals that her BUN and serum creatinine are slightly elevated and that she has 2+ protein and 1+ RBC in her urine.

4. Of what significance are these findings, and what is the relationship of such findings to D.W.'s diagnosis of SLE?

5. How will D.W.'s treatment and nursing plan likely change?

D.W. is seen in the immunology clinic twice monthly during the next 3 months. Although her condition does not worsen, her BUN and serum creatinine remain elevated. While at work one afternoon, D.W. begins to feel dizzy and develops a severe headache. She reports to her supervisor who has her lie down. When D.W. starts to become disoriented, her supervisor calls 911, and D.W. is taken to the hospital. D.W. is admitted for probable lupus cerebritis r/t acute exacerbation of her disease.

6. What preventive measures should be instituted to protect D.W. at this time?

7. What additional problems indicative of CNS involvement r/t SLE should D.W. be assessed for?

D.W. is again placed on IV methylprednisolone and started on plasmapheresis.

8. What major complications associated with immunosuppression therapy will D.W. have to be monitored for?

9. What does plasmapheresis do, and why might it reduce the s/s associated with SLE?

10. What data would support the assumption that D.W.'s condition is stabilizing?

11. Identify at least five topics that D.W. must be taught before she is discharged that may help her lead as normal a life as possible.

12. You note that D.W.'s husband is visiting her this afternoon. You enter the room to ask whether they have any questions. D.W.'s husband states, "I have tried to tell her that she cannot go back to work. Sure, we need the money, but the kids and I need her more. I'm afraid that this lupus has weakened her whole body and it will kill her if she goes back to work. Is that right?" How would you respond to his concerns?

Additional information on SLE can be found through the following resources:

http://www.nlm.nih.gov/medlineplus/lupus.html

http://www.nih.gov/niams/ (National Institute of Arthritis and Musculoskeletal and Skin Diseases)

Bonus Project: Locate and print a patient education handout on SLE in both English and Spanish. Atttach it to this assignment.

Oncologic/Hematologic Disorders

Case Study 1

Name ______________________ Class/Group ______ Date ______

Group Members ____

INSTRUCTIONS: All questions apply to this case study. Your responses should be brief and to the point. Adequate space has been provided for answers. When asked to provide several answers, they should be listed in order of priority or significance. Do not assume information that is not provided. Please print or write clearly. If your response is not legible, it will be marked as ? and you will need to rewrite it.

Scenario

B.B., a 53-year-old divorced professional woman, was diagnosed with stage T1 N0 M0 infiltrating ductal breast cancer on her right side based on a lumpectomy and axillary lymph node dissection over a year ago. After her radiation therapy (daily treatments for 6 weeks) was completed, she was placed on tamoxifen (to be taken for five years). She has been coming to the clinic every 3 months for her checkup in the year since her treatment was completed. In addition to working at the clinic, you are a volunteer consultant to the Encore-YWCA support group for women who have had breast cancer, where B.B. regularly attends. The group has invited you to present "Breast Cancer: Prevention, Screening, and Detection Guidelines" at their next meeting.

1. What is tamoxifen? Why are women placed on long-term tamoxifen therapy as a treatment for breast cancer?

2. What is an axillary lymph node dissection? Why did B.B. have an axillary lymph node dissection with her lumpectomy?

3. B.B. was diagnosed with stage T1 N0 M0 breast cancer. What does that mean?

4. What risk factors for breast cancer will you include in your group presentation? ❍ ❍ ❍ ❍ ❍

5. What will you teach the group about early detection of breast cancer? ❍ ❍ ❍ ❍ ❍

6. What educational equipment can help women learn how to perform BSE correctly and how to detect lumps? ❍ ❍ ❍ ❍ ❍

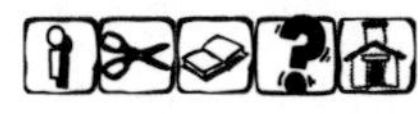

7. Describe the technique for performing BSE correctly. ❍ ❍ ❍ ❍ ❍

8. One of the women in the group shows you how the arm on the side that had the breast cancer is more swollen than the other arm. She said she is having a lot of trouble with this. What do you think is happening? How will you explain this to her? What will you advise her? ❍ ❍ ❍ ❍ ❍

9. B.B. raises her hand and tells you she heard she should never have her BP taken in her affected arm (the right arm in her case). You remember that you told her this in the office, but you realize she was probably too anxious or tired to remember exactly what you said. What will you advise her and the other women present? ❍ ❍ ❍ ❍ ❍

10. B.B. also says she was told to watch for infection in her affected arm. She asks why that's important. What will you tell her? ❍ ❍ ❍ ❍ ❍

11. What are some other things breast cancer survivors can do to manage or prevent lymphedema? (List four.)

For more information on risk factors, consult the following resources:

The Department of Defense Breast Cancer Decision Guide
https://www.bcdg.org/

American Cancer Society
1599 Clifton Road, N.E.
Atlanta, GA 30329-4251
Telephone: (800) ACS-2345
http://www.cancer.org

National Cancer Institute (NCI)
Building 31, Room 10A03
31 Center Drive, MSC 2580
Bethesda, MD 20892-2580
www.nci.nih.gov

National Cancer Information Service
Telephone: (800) 4-CANCER

Case Study 2

Name ____________________ Class/Group ______ Date ______

Group Members ______________________________

INSTRUCTIONS: All questions apply to this case study. Your responses should be brief and to the point. Adequate space has been provided for answers. When asked to provide several answers, they should be listed in order of priority or significance. Do not assume information that is not provided. Please print or write clearly. If your response is not legible, it will be marked as ? and you will need to rewrite it.

❍ ❍ ❍ / ❍ ❍

Scenario

V.M. is a 39-year-old black man who has sickle cell disease (SCD), sometimes called sickle cell anemia, marked by frequent episodes of severe pain. His anemia has been managed with multiple transfusions, and he shows signs of chronic renal failure. He is a nonsmoker, nondrinker, and is on social security disability. His regular medications are pentoxifylline (Trental), oxycodone/acetaminophen (Roxicet), and folic acid (Folvite). In hematology clinic this AM, V.M.'s Hgb measured 6.7 g/dL. He received 2 units packed red cells (PRC) over 3 hours and then went home. He developed dyspnea and SOB approximately 1 to 1½ hours later, and his wife called 911. The emergency medical system (EMS) crew initiated oxygen and transported V.M. to the ED.

1. What is sickle cell disease, and how is it r/t race? ❍ ❍ ❍ ❍ ❍

2. The stiff, sickled RBC tends to cause vascular occlusions with subsequent local infarction. As a rule, the spleen suffers so many vasoocclusive/infarction episodes that it is greatly reduced in size and is rendered nonfunctional by the time the individual is 6 years of age. What are the implications of having a nonfunctioning spleen? ❍ ❍ ❍ ❍ ❍

3. Identify two mechanisms that contribute to anemia in patients with SCD. ❍ ❍ ❍ ❍ ❍

4. On arrival to the ED, the physician asks V.M. if he is in pain and if he needs Demerol. V.M. answers "No" to both questions. Why did the physician ask these two questions?

5. V.M.'s ABGs on 9 L O_2/simple face mask are pH 7.34, PaO_2 74 mm Hg, $PaCO_2$ 33 mm Hg, HCO_3 18 mEq/L, BE –6. Is V.M. being adequately oxygenated? Why or why not?

6. V.M. c/o being SOB. Do you believe his low Hgb level is responsible for his complaints?

You perform a quick assessment and note a systolic murmur and crackles in V.M.'s bases bilaterally. VS are 176/102, 94, 28, 97° F (oral). As you start an IV, you draw blood for hemogram with differential, basic metabolic panel, calcium, and phosphorous and send it for analysis.

7. Your assessment findings are consistent with fluid overload. What four findings led you to that conclusion?

8. What action would you expect the physician to take next, and why?

The lab values return: Na 137 mmol/L, K 4.9 mmol/L, Cl 110 mmol/L, CO_2 16 mmol/L, BUN 27 mg/dL, creatinine 2.7 mg/dL, Ca 8.2 mg/dL, PO_4 4.7 mg/dL, WBC 4.3 thou/cmm, Hgb 7.8 g/dL, Hct 20.9%, platelets 208 thou/cmm.

9. What is the significance of the lab results, and why?

The physician prescribes furosemide (Lasix) 20 mg IVP now, methylprednisolone (Solu-Medrol) 125 mg IVP, and ceftriaxone (Rocephin) 1 g IVPB after the Lasix.

10. Explain the significance of using each of these drugs.

11. Why is it difficult to cross-match blood to transfuse V.M.?

As V.M.'s SOB is relieved, he shakes the physician's hand and thanks him for asking about the presence of pain and the need for pain medication. V.M. states, "One of my biggest fears is that I'll come here in crisis and the doctor won't treat my pain aggressively enough. I don't want to be labeled as a drug seeker or an emergency room abuser."

12. Why would V.M. be concerned about obtaining adequate pain control in the ED?

V.M. voids 1900 ml within 2 hours of the Lasix administration. On repeat assessment, the systolic murmur is audible, but all lung fields are clear. Repeat VS are 160/94, 82, 20, 98° F (oral). V.M. is discharged to home on his previous medications.

13. What issues would you address with V.M. before he is discharged?

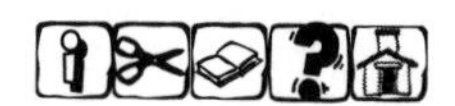

For more information contact:
Comprehensive Sickle Cell Centers
http://www.rhofed.com/sickle/

Case Study 3

Name ____________________ Class/Group ______ Date ______

Group Members ____________________

INSTRUCTIONS: All questions apply to this case study. Your responses should be brief and to the point. Adequate space has been provided for answers. When asked to provide several answers, they should be listed in order of priority or significance. Do not assume information that is not provided. Please print or write clearly. If your response is not legible, it will be marked as ? and you will need to rewrite it.

Scenario

D.M. is a married 36-year-old woman with 4 children who works part-time as a clerk. She is 5'8" tall and weighs 135 lb. She has insurance through her husband's employer. She has never smoked and has an occasional social drink. She has PMH of plastic surgery for breast implants in August of last year. When she returned for her breast implant check-up 10 months later, a 2.2-cm lump was discovered in her R breast. When a biopsy indicated the lump was malignant, she elected to have a lumpectomy and axillary lymph node dissection. The pathology report indicated that 3 of 14 lymph nodes were positive. Her CT scan and bone scans were negative. You are a staff nurse at the group oncology clinic where she was referred to receive chemotherapy. After she completes chemotherapy, she is scheduled to receive radiation therapy. Admitting diagnosis: infiltrating ductal carcinoma, stage T2 N1 M0, premenopausal, estrogen receptor 3+, progesterone neg, and Her2-neu 3+. (Note: Her2-neu is also known as C-ErbB-2)

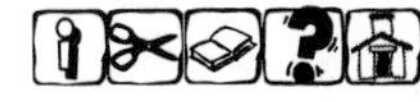

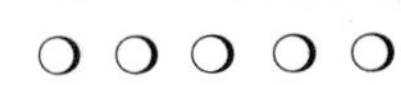

1. D.M. wants you to explain exactly what stage T2 N1 M0 means. What will you tell her?

2. Next, D.M. wants to know what the ER, PR, and Her2-neu values mean.

3. She asks you to explain what her chances of survival are. How will you explain this to her? ❍ ❍ ❍ ❍ ❍

4. D.M. will be receiving 6 cycles of combination chemotherapy, consisting of doxirubicin (Adriamycin), and cyclophosphamide (Cytoxan). What are the major side effects you want to prepare her for? ❍ ❍ ❍ ❍ ❍

5. Elaborate on issues r/t head/hair care. ❍ ❍ ❍ ❍ ❍

6. What is a major complication in patients receiving a high amount of Adriamycin? ❍ ❍ ❍ ❍ ❍

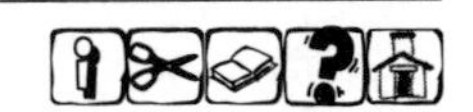

7. Explain to D.M. in lay terms what she needs to know about immunosuppression. ❍ ❍ ❍ ❍ ❍

D.M. completes her chemotherapy. She lost most of her hair and has been wearing a scarf but now her hair is beginning to grow back. She is being transferred to the radiation therapy department for treatment and is scheduled to begin radiation therapy.

You perform an admission assessment. Findings are as follows: Wt. 148 lb; VS 104/70, 80, 20, 98.0° F (oral). Cardiovascular: S_1 S_2 without murmurs or rubs. Respiratory: clear to auscultation throughout. Neuromuscular/skeletal: negative, patient c/o of fatigue, no c/o bone pain. GI: without hepatosplenomegaly or masses. GU: negative. Integumentary/oral: hair growth 1/4" over entire head, oral mucosa reddened, and patient c/o soreness. Lymph node: no palpable adenopathy in the cervical, supraclavicular, axillary, or inguinal nodes.

8. What areas of the above assessment concern you? Explain. ❍ ❍ ❍ ❍ ❍

D.M. receives 6 weeks of daily (weekdays) radiation therapy treatments with a total dose of 6400 cGy. She has a terrible time with fatigue, and at one point tells you, "When I lie down, I can't become enough of the bed!" You helped her develop an activity-rest plan and support her in obtaining outside help with housework. At her last visit, she tells you, "Now I hope I can see my kids grow up." She is scheduled to return to the oncologist every 3 months for follow-up care and monitoring.

9. D.M. comes to her scheduled follow-up appointment. She appears very anxious. When questioned, she tells you, "I've been worried about my daughters. What if they get breast cancer? What can I do to help them?" What is your response?

10. You ask her whether she has other questions. She tells you she is worried about the breast cancer coming back and wants to know whether she would have to go through the chemotherapy and radiation therapy all over again. What can you do, and what will you tell her?

D.M. seems to do fine for a while. On her 9-month follow-up visit, she tells you she has been having headaches for the past few weeks. Her MRI indicates she has metastases to the brain. She undergoes a bone marrow transplant; unfortunately, it fails to stop her cancer. She dies at the age of 38, leaving behind 4 children, ages 4 through 14.

Case Study 4

Name ______________________ Class/Group ______ Date ______

Group Members ______________________________________

INSTRUCTIONS: All questions apply to this case study. Your responses should be brief and to the point. Adequate space has been provided for answers. When asked to provide several answers, they should be listed in order of priority or significance. Do not assume information that is not provided. Please print or write clearly. If your response is not legible, it will be marked as ? and you will need to rewrite it.

❍ ❍ ❍ / ❍ ❍

Scenario

A.V. is a 37-year-old married housewife with a 35 pack-year history of smoking. She says she "just can't quit." She denies ETOH use. Ht 5'7" Wt 115 lb. Her PMH includes C-sections for all 3 children ages 6, 14, and 18. She does not have insurance. She noticed a "canker sore" on the anterior lateral aspect of her L tongue several months ago. Over time, she developed a sore throat and ear pain. The family nurse practitioner at the low-income clinic sent her to a specialist who performed a biopsy of her anterior tongue. The diagnosis was squamous cell carcinoma poorly differentiated T2 N0. Before her surgery she had complete panoramic views of her mandible; fluoride trays were made followed by a partial glossectomy and excision of the floor of her mouth. Three weeks after surgery, multiple teeth are scheduled to be extracted. Afterward, she will be scheduled for 8 weeks of radiation therapy in your outpatient clinic.

1. Describe the rationale for this prophylactic treatment: teeth extraction, panoramic views, fluoride trays. ❍ ❍ ❍ ❍ ❍

2. Identify and describe preop nursing care for partial glossectomy. ❍ ❍ ❍ ❍ ❍

3. Identify and describe potential postop care for partial glossectomy.

4. Identify and describe potential postop complications resulting from a partial glossectomy. Plan appropriate nursing interventions and patient teaching strategies to manage these complications.

5. When she returns for her first postop visit to your clinic, she appears to be quite distressed to hear about the radiation therapy. Although she still has considerable trouble speaking, she explains she really didn't think much about it before surgery. She seems quite embarrassed as she tells you her family has no insurance, and they were barely making it earlier. Now she says she is getting "nasty letters" from the hospital demanding payment. What can you do?

6. As she sits by you, she keeps her hand over her mouth and jaw. She is wearing her hair so that it hangs down over her face. Her jaw and neck still are swollen from the surgery and tooth extraction. She avoids eye contact with you. How will you respond?

Case Study 5

Name ______________________ Class/Group ______ Date ______

Group Members ____________________________________

INSTRUCTIONS: All questions apply to this case study. Your responses should be brief and to the point. Adequate space has been provided for answers. When asked to provide several answers, they should be listed in order of priority or significance. Do not assume information that is not provided. Please print or write clearly. If your response is not legible, it will be marked as ? and you will need to rewrite it.

Scenario

A.T. is a 21-year-old college student. He works part-time as a manual laborer, uses half a can of smokeless tobacco each week, and drinks a 6-pack of beer on the weekend. A year ago in September, he discovered a small, painless lump in his lower L neck. Over the quarter, he experienced increasing fatigue and a 10-lb weight loss that he attributed to "working and studying too hard." In the spring, he saw a nurse practitioner at the student health center who immediately referred him to an oncologist. A lymph node biopsy revealed Hodgkin's disease. The gallium scan, bone scan, and CT scan of the chest, abdomen, and pelvis all came back negative. A staging laparotomy was conducted a month later to confirm the diagnosis. His diagnosis was Hodgkin's disease, stage IA, mixed cellularity. You are a staff nurse in the outpatient oncology services when A.T. comes in.

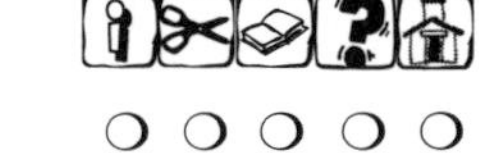

1. A.T. wants to know what Hodgkin's disease is and how he "caught" it. What will you tell him?

2. A.T. wants to know what "stage IA" means; he also wants to know the significance of the test results. What are you going to tell him?

A few days later, you see A.T. in the oncologist's office during his appointment to discuss the treatment regimen for radiation therapy. His prescribed radiation treatment regimen (outpatient) includes Monday through Friday with treatments scheduled for approximately 6 to 10 weeks. Admission assessment findings on his first visit to the outpatient oncology clinic at the end of January are Wt 183 lb, Ht 78 in. VS 124/66, 60, 16, 98.0° F (oral). Cardiovascular: heart rate regular. Respiratory: clear to auscultation. Neuromuscular/skeletal, GI, and GU: negative. Integumentary/oral: incision from staging laparotomy well-approximated without erythema, edema, pain, or drainage. Incision from lymph node dissection healing well, oral mucosa pink and moist, no palpable adenopathy.

3. What abnormal assessment findings do you recognize in the previous information? ❍ ❍ ❍ ❍ ❍

4. A.T. jokes with you that he's "going to get nuked and glow." What information would you include in your teaching to prepare him for radiation treatments? ❍ ❍ ❍ ❍ ❍

5. You have developed a good relationship with A.T. during the multiple visits required for his radiation therapy. He shares some futuristic goals and says, "What are the chances that I will beat this cancer?" Respond to A.T.'s request. ❍ ❍ ❍ ❍ ❍

Other kinds of cancer may occur many years later as a result of the toxic effects of earlier treatment. This is one reason why cancer specialists are reluctant to use the word "cured."

6. What other issues of survivorship may affect patients like A.T. (e.g., insurance, employability)? ❍ ❍ ❍ ❍ ❍

7. How and what are you going to counsel and teach A.J. about potential sterility/infertility side effects of treatment? ❍ ❍ ❍ ❍ ❍

8. Six weeks into therapy, A.T. drags himself into the clinic one Friday, drops into a chair, and wearily states, "I'm quitting. If this is what life is like, it's not worth living." How would you respond to him? ❍ ❍ ❍ ❍ ❍

9. When A.T. checks in this week, he weighs 177 lb. When you express concern, he tells you he just doesn't have any appetite. How are you going to respond? List at least four interventions.

10. At his final appointment, A.T.'s laboratory values are WBC 3.3 thou/cmm, Hgb 14 g/dl, Hct 41%, and platelets 369 thou/cmm. His VS are 120/76, 84, 20, 98.0° F(oral). Wt 175 lb. Do any of these values concern you? Explain.

A.T. is discharged from radiation and scheduled to see an oncologist every three months for follow-up care.

Case Study 6

Name ______________________ Class/Group ______ Date ______

Group Members ____

INSTRUCTIONS: All questions apply to this case study. Your responses should be brief and to the point. Adequate space has been provided for answers. When asked to provide several answers, they should be listed in order of priority or significance. Do not assume information that is not provided. Please print or write clearly. If your response is not legible, it will be marked as ? and you will need to rewrite it.

❍ ❍ ❍ / ❍ ❍

Scenario

C.W. is a 42-year-old divorced woman with adenocarcinoma (cancer) of the lung with metastasis (spread) to the brain and liver. She is the single parent of a 17-year-old son, has experienced episodic health care, is currently unemployed because of poor health, and has no health insurance. She has smoked 1 to 2 packs per day for 20 years. PMH includes cholecystectomy, hysterectomy, and breast augmentation. In May of last year, she developed scapular and arm pain in her right side, was diagnosed with adenocarcinoma of the lung, and underwent a wedge resection of the upper right lobe of the lung. Because she had no insurance, she did not receive follow-up care (e.g., radiation therapy and/or chemotherapy).

C.W. developed pain in her right temple 48 hours ago and was seen in the ED, where she was given cephradine (Velosef). C.W. had a seizure 24 hours later, was transported to the ED, and was diagnosed as having an allergic reaction to the Velosef. She was instructed to call her family doctor. C.W.'s doctor was unavailable for 48 hours. After suffering a tonic-clonic (grand mal) seizure at home, she was admitted to a rural hospital. A CT scan revealed a large mass in the right frontal area of her brain. Dexamethasone (Decadron) was given IV, and an oncologist in the metropolitan area was consulted. C.W. was transferred to your oncology unit postseizure with slightly slurred speech and intermittent bone pain. She has lost 22 lb in the past year. She is receiving acetaminophen/hydrocodone (Lortab) 1 to 2 5-mg tabs every 3 to 4 hours, as needed. C.W.'s record lists codeine and milk allergies.

1. Identify the usual location, growth rate, and likelihood of metastasis of adenocarcinoma of the lung. ❍ ❍ ❍ ❍ ❍

2. Is the presence of bone pain and weight loss significant? ❍ ❍ ❍ ❍ ❍

3. What tests are likely to be performed to determine whether C.W.'s adenocarcinoma has metastasized? ❍ ❍ ❍ ❍ ❍

4. The tests are performed, and C.W. is diagnosed with adenocarcinoma of the lung with metastasis to lymph nodes, liver, and brain. She is scheduled to receive 10 radiation therapy treatments to the whole brain (3 as an inpatient, 7 as an outpatient). Identify five needs that you will address with C.W. and her son.

After her third radiation treatment, C.W. is discharged on the following medications: dexamethasone 4 mg PO q8h; propoxyphene/acetaminophen (Darvocet-N) 100 mg PO q4h prn; prochloperazine maleate (Compazine spansules) 15 mg PO q12h prn; temazepam 30 mg PO this prn.

5. What is the rationale for C.W. receiving each medication?

Two months post-hospital discharge and follow-up therapy, C.W. continues to have increasing symptoms of pain, anorexia, weight loss, edema in extremities, and insomnia. Her son accompanied her to the physician's office. While his mother is having her blood drawn, he asks the nurse what is going to happen to his mother.

6. How would you respond to him?

7. He asks what he can do to help his mother. What information could you give him? ❍ ❍ ❍ ❍ ❍

8. As C.W.'s disease progresses, what s/s can be anticipated, and what kind of relief can be provided? ❍ ❍ ❍ ❍ ❍

9. C.W.'s son says he's never been around someone who is dying before. He expresses fear he won't know what to do. How can you help him? ❍ ❍ ❍ ❍ ❍

Case Study 7

Name ______________________ Class/Group ______ Date ______

Group Members ____

INSTRUCTIONS: All questions apply to this case study. Your responses should be brief and to the point. Adequate space has been provided for answers. When asked to provide several answers, they should be listed in order of priority or significance. Do not assume information that is not provided. Please print or write clearly. If your response is not legible, it will be marked as ? and you will need to rewrite it.

❍ ❍ ❍ / ❍ ❍

Scenario

D.L., a 21-year-old single man who works as a plumber's assistant, developed low back pain "from a work injury" 2 weeks ago. He had no PMH and is a nonsmoker, nondrinker. He is instructed to take diclofenac (Voltaren) 50 mg PO tid for 6 doses and cyclobenzaprine (Flexeril) 10 mg PO tid for 6 doses. Within 2 to 3 days, he develops a fever (101.6° F, oral), and a rash develops over his entire body. He shows dramatic bruising; he also develops a decreased appetite and a sore mouth. He is taken to the ER at a rural hospital when he starts vomiting blood. His labs are WBC 31.7 thou/cmm, Hgb 10.1 g/dL, Hct 29%, and platelets 16 thou/cmm. Arrangements are made to transfer him to the regional medical center (where you work on the heme/onc unit) to see an oncologist for a workup and to be admitted to the hospital for therapy. A bone marrow biopsy confirms the diagnosis of acute lymphoblastic leukemia (ALL).

1. What is ALL, and what are other names for this same condition? ❍ ❍ ❍ ❍ ❍

2. You are the leukemia support and education group leader for your hospital. Patients attending your sessions have acute/chronic lymphocytic leukemia, acute/chronic myelogenous leukemia, myelodysplastic syndrome, and multiple myeloma. Your topic for discussion today is the etiology of these oncologic/hematologic disorders. D.L.'s older brother, T.L., is a nursing student, and he wants to know how many kinds of leukemia there are and if they are caused by the same thing. List the related diseases in the leukemia family and what is thought to cause each. ❍ ❍ ❍ ❍ ❍

3. D.L. asks you what the chances are for someone, like him, with ALL. What can you tell him?

D.L. is scheduled to receive the initial induction combination chemotherapy by IV and IT (intrathecal) routes. He will be receiving doxorubicin, vincristine and cyclophosphamide IVP, methotrexate IT, and prednisone PO. He will be hospitalized about 3 weeks. He will be scheduled for intense consolidation courses, and then maintenance therapy for 1 year. The induction and consolidation courses are intense drug therapies, requiring multiple blood product infusions and antibiotic therapy to aid recovery. Because of his projected required course of therapy, he will be unable to work and will probably lose his insurance.

D.L.'s admission assessments are as follows: VS 140/74, 90, 24, 103.3° F (oral). Wt 150 lb. Cardiovascular: normal sinus rhythm, no S_3, S_4 rubs, or murmurs, all peripheral pulses present. Respiratory: clear to auscultation. Neuromuscular/skeletal: grossly intact. Motor and sensory exam normal. GI: Spleen about 5 fingerbreadths below the right costal margin-tender; liver is not enlarged; no ascites or intraabdominal mass or CVA tenderness. GU: rectal not done. Integumentary/oral: HEENT, nomocephalic, pupils level, round, reactive to light in accommodation; no sclera icterus; conjunctiva very pale; fundoscopic exam benign; oropharynx has some gingival lesions; mucous membranes moist and pale; tympanic membranes normal; neck supple; trachea midline; thyroid normal; no murmurs or JVD distention. To facilitate D.L.'s chemotherapy and blood product infusion, a triple-lumen subclavian catheter is inserted.

4. Describe potential effects the acute leukemia, treatment, and rehabilitation have on the socioeconomic status and family relationships of people like D.L.

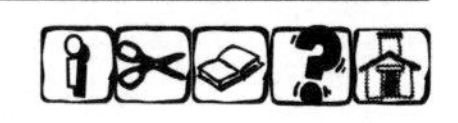

5. During the next 14 days, D.L. receives irradiated platelets and leukoreduced, irradiated RBCs. What is the rationale for using irradiated, leukoreduced blood products? Describe the nursing administration/monitoring procedure for these products. ❍ ❍ ❍ ❍ ❍

6. D.L. will continue to receive intense combination chemotherapy for several more weeks. Because of limited finances, his hospitalization stay will be cut short. What are the major self-care management issues for home care that need to be reinforced?

7. D.L. is going to be staying with his parents. T.L. has promised to help with D.L.'s care. In addition, a home care nurse will visit him twice weekly. You are going to teach D.L. and his brother, T.L., to care for and use his triple-lumen subclavian catheter. What will you tell them?

Before he leaves, T.L. says, "You know, I've been studying about some of this stuff in my med-surg class, but I had no idea how bad it feels to go through this. I hope this makes me a better, more sensitive nurse."

Case Study 8

Name ______________________ Class/Group ______ Date ______

Group Members ______________________________________

INSTRUCTIONS: All questions apply to this case study. Your responses should be brief and to the point. Adequate space has been provided for answers. When asked to provide several answers, they should be listed in order of priority or significance. Do not assume information that is not provided. Please print or write clearly. If your response is not legible, it will be marked as ? and you will need to rewrite it.

❍ ❍ ❍ / ❍ ❍

Scenario

C.P. is a 71-year-old married farmer, with a PMH of hernia surgery in 1965 and prostate surgery in 1992 for BPH (benign prostatic hyperplasia). C.P. does not drink but he has smoked for 40 years; the past 3 years he has smoked 2 to 3 packs per day. He has no known allergies. Six months ago, C.P. visited the local rural health clinic with c/o progressive cough and chest congestion. Despite a week of antibiotic therapy, C.P. continued to worsen; he experienced progressive dyspnea and productive cough, and he began to have night sweats. C.P. refuses to be admitted to the hospital ("There's no one to look after the cows") but agrees to go for a CXR. His insurance company also insists on this being done on an out-patient basis. The radiologist reads C.P.'s CXR as left hilar lung mass, probable lung cancer. C.P. is scheduled for a diagnostic fiberoptic bronchoscopy with endobronchial lung biopsy as an outpatient to confirm the diagnosis.

1. What is fiberoptic bronchoscopy? What information will a fiberoptic bronchoscopy with endobronchial lung biopsy provide? ❍ ❍ ❍ ❍ ❍

2. As the nurse who works with the pulmonologist, it is your responsibility to prepare C.P. for the fiberoptic bronchoscopy procedure. What would you include in your teaching plan? ❍ ❍ ❍ ❍ ❍

3. What is your responsibility during and immediately after the bronchoscopy? ❍ ❍ ❍ ❍ ❍

4. C.P. tolerates the procedure well. He returns to the office in 4 days to learn the results of his test. The pulmonologist tells C.P. and his wife that he has oat cell lung cancer and explains that it is a very fast-growing cancer with a poor prognosis. This kind of lung cancer is directly r/t C.P.'s history of smoking. What is your role at this time? ❍ ❍ ❍ ❍ ❍

C.P. is scheduled to begin combination chemotherapy with cisplatin (Platinol) and etoposide (VePesid). He plans to continue to work the farm as long as possible; his brother-in-law has promised to help him.

5. How would you explain combination chemotherapy and how it works to C.P. and his wife? ❍ ❍ ❍ ❍ ❍

6. C.P.'s wife tells you she's heard that chemotherapy makes you really sick. How would you explain chemotherapy side effects? ❍ ❍ ❍ ❍ ❍

7. What are the most common side effects of cisplatin and VePesid? ❍ ❍ ❍ ❍ ❍

8. Based on your knowledge of the most common side effects, list at least seven interventions that should be incorporated into his plan of care?

9. C.P. needs to have a working understanding of how to balance his treatments with his work. You sit down with C.P. to plan a daily work/activity/rest schedule to accommodate his treatments and side effects. List at least four concepts you would emphasize.

10. C.P. receives cisplatin 60 mg in 100-ml NS IV over 1 to 2 hours daily, the first 3 days of each month for 6 months, and VePesid 200 mg in 250-ml NS IV over 1 to 2 hours daily, the first 3 days of each month for 6 months. What is the nadir for each drug, and what implications does the nadir have for C.P.?

A month later, when C.P. returns for his second round of chemotherapy, he c/o SOB, chest tightness, and palpitations. He looks exhausted. ECG and CXR reveal A fib and LLL pneumonia with L pleural effusion. C.P. is admitted to the hospital with the following laboratory values: WBC 2.5 thou/cmm, RBC 5.6 thou/cmm, Hgb 17.7 g/dL, Hct 51.7%, platelets 252.0 thou/cmm, PT/INR ratio 8.8, PTT 29.7 sec, Na 131 mmol/L, K 4.2 mmol/L, Cl 90 mmol/L, CO_2 25 mEq/L, BUN 13 mg/dL, creatinine 0.8 mg/dL, glucose 175 mg/dL.

11. What do these lab values indicate?

12. The pulmonologist performs a thoracentesis and prescribes cefotaximine 1 g IV and q8h erythromycin 500 mg IV q6h. What factor in C.P.'s background will complicate his diagnosis of pneumonia?

13. C.P.'s condition continues to deteriorate. He tells you he doesn't want to live like this, but the doctor wants to continue with aggressive therapy. Discuss the pros and cons of continued therapy and what role you can play in helping him.

C.P. is given the second round of chemotherapy and is discharged to home. He receives no further treatment and dies 2 weeks later.

Case Study 9

Name ______________________ Class/Group ______ Date ______

Group Members ______________________________________

INSTRUCTIONS: All questions apply to this case study. Your responses should be brief and to the point. Adequate space has been provided for answers. When asked to provide several answers, they should be listed in order of priority or significance. Do not assume information that is not provided. Please print or write clearly. If your response is not legible, it will be marked as ? and you will need to rewrite it.

❍ ❍ ❍ / ❍ ❍

Scenario

You are caring for J.B., a 56-year-old woman with colon cancer. PMH includes colon resection followed by combined chemotherapy approximately 18 months ago; recently diagnosed with recurrence of colon cancer; chemotherapy was administered for 5 of the 8 scheduled cycles; previous significant weight loss (current Ht 67", Wt 105 lb); 50 pack-year (2 PPD x 25 yr) smoking history. J.B. is admitted for acute N/V and dehydration. She is nutritionally depleted. Her physician determines that diagnostic evaluation requires exploratory laparotomy. VS 150/90, 124, 26, 100° F.

1. List at least five major risks and potential complications for J.B.? ❍ ❍ ❍ ❍ ❍

2. The physician performs an exploratory laparotomy for lysis of adhesions, small bowel resection, colectomy, and colostomy with Hartman's pouch. After surgery, J.B. is admitted to the SICU with a large abdominal dressing. You roll J.B. side-to-side to remove the soiled surgical linen, and the dressing becomes saturated with a large amount of serosanguinous drainage. Would the drainage be expected after abdominal surgery? Explain. ❍ ❍ ❍ ❍ ❍

3. Traditionally, the physician performs the first dressing change. Why is this done?

4. The physician removes the surgical dressing. The wound edges are well approximated, the suture line is edematous, the staples are intact, the transverse colostomy rosebud looks pink in the middle and dark around the edges, and there are two Jackson-Pratt drains in the RMQ. Do any of these findings concern you, and why?

The physician prescribes the following TPN orders: amino acids 10% 100 ml; dextrose 70%, 1000 ml; water for injection 1000 ml; sodium acetate 20 mEq; sodium phosphate 20 mEq; potassium acetate 20 mEq; KCl 90 mEq; calcium gluconate 20 mEq; magnesium sulfate 10 mEq; regular insulin 10 units; multivitamins 1 amp; heparin 1200 units. Infuse 3000 ml volume over 24h daily.

5. List and explain at least five nursing management activities you should provide to minimize the potential side effects for J.B.

6. The TPN infusion is complete, the alarm is sounding, and the pharmacy has not delivered the next bottle of TPN. What action should you take, and why?

7. Within minutes of sitting in the chair, you note that J.B. is becoming increasingly pale and diaphoretic. Her pulse is rapid and irregular and she c/o being nauseated and dizzy. What actions should you take next?

8. J.B. looks at you and tells you that she knows she is never going to leave the hospital alive. She says she has a lot of regrets. She confides that she used to drink a lot and wasn't a good mother to her 3 children; her son hasn't spoken to her in 15 years. How should you respond?

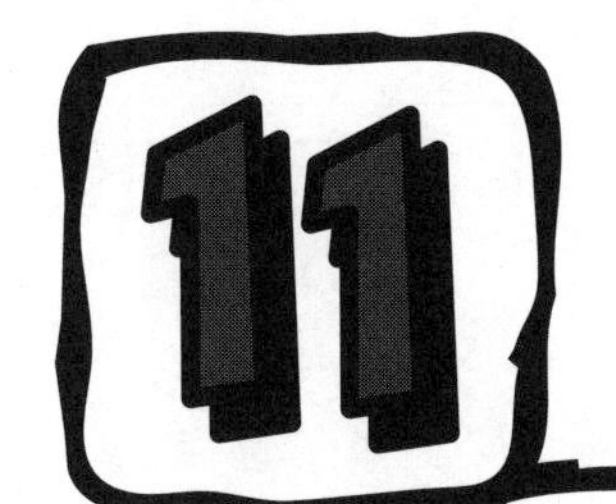

Multiple System Disorders

Case Study 1

Name ______________________ Class/Group ______ Date ______

Group Members ______________________________________

INSTRUCTIONS: All questions apply to this case study. Your responses should be brief and to the point. Adequate space has been provided for answers. When asked to provide several answers, they should be listed in order of priority or significance. Do not assume information that is not provided. Please print or write clearly. If your response is not legible, it will be marked as ? and you will need to rewrite it.

Scenario

You are working the day shift on the medical-surgical unit in a small, rural community hospital. Your assignment includes an 18-year-old woman, A.N., admitted at night. A.N. was burned in a house fire and sustained burns over 30% of body surface area, with partial-thickness burns on her legs and back.

1. A.N. is undergoing burn fluid resuscitation using the standard Baxter (Parkland) formula. She was burned at 0200 and admitted at 0400. She weighs 110 lb. Calculate her fluid requirements, and specify how much will be given and what time intervals will be used.

2. A.N. was sleeping when the fire started and managed to make her way out of the house through thick smoke. You are concerned about possible smoke inhalation. What assessment findings would corroborate this concern?

3. A.N. is very concerned about visible scars. What will you tell her to allay her fears?

4. A.N. is in severe pain. What is the drug of choice for pain relief following burn injury, and how should it be given?

5. A.N.'s burns are to be treated by the open method with topical application of silver sufadiazine (Silvadene). What is the major drawback to this method of treatment?

6. A special burn diet is ordered for A.N.. She has always gained weight easily and is concerned about the size of the portions. What diet-related teaching will you provide?

7. Tissues under and around A.N.'s burns are severely swollen. She looks at you with tears in her eyes and asks, "Will they stay this way?" What is your answer?

8. Following significant burn injury, the patient is at high risk for infection. What nursing measures will you institute to prevent this?

9. A.N. has one area of circumferential burns on her right lower leg. What complication is she in danger of developing, and how will you monitor for it?

Case Study 2

Name ______________________ Class/Group ______ Date ______

Group Members ______________________________

INSTRUCTIONS: All questions apply to this case study. Your responses should be brief and to the point. Adequate space has been provided for answers. When asked to provide several answers, they should be listed in order of priority or significance. Do not assume information that is not provided. Please print or write clearly. If your response is not legible, it will be marked as ? and you will need to rewrite it.

Scenario

You are working evenings on an orthopedic floor. One of your patients, J.O., is a 25-year-old man who was a new admission on day shift. He was involved in a motor vehicle accident (MVA) during a high-speed police chase. His admitting diagnosis is status post (s/p) open reduction and internal ORIF of the R femur (which was performed under general anesthesia), multiple rib fractures, sternal bruise, and multiple abrasions. He speaks some English but is more comfortable with his "home" language. He is under arrest for narcotics trafficking, so one wrist is shackled to the bed and he has a guard with him continuously. Another drug dealer has told him "he's coming to get him." Hospital security is aware of the situation.

Your initial assessment reveals stable VS of 116/78, 84, 16, 98.6° F. His only complaint is pain, for which he has a PCA pump. He has crackles in lung bases bilaterally. His abdomen is soft and nontender. He has an indwelling Foley catheter and an nasogastric tube connected to low wall suction. His IV of D_5LR is infusing in the proximal port of a L subclavian triple lumen catheter; the remaining two ports are heparin-locked. His R femur is connected to skeletal traction. The dressing is dry and intact over the incision site.

1. J.O. wants to smoke a cigarette. He usually smokes a pack a day and has had none since the accident. He is irate because the day nurse would not let him smoke. What is your major concern about J.O.'s smoking?

2. Do you think J.O. would be a good candidate for a nicotine patch? Why or why not? State your rationale.

3. J.O.'s right leg is connected to 10 pounds of skeletal traction. As you troubleshoot the system, you note that the ropes are knotted at connection sites, the pulleys have rope running along the center tracts, the leg is slightly flexed at the knee, the leg is 6 inches above the mattress, and the 10-pound weight is resting on the floor. Are any of these findings of concern to you? If so, how would you fix it?

The nurse in the ED phones to tell you that J.O.'s immunization status could not be determined when he arrived so no tetanus immunization was given. When you ask J.O. the date of his last tetanus shot, he looks puzzled and asks you what a tetanus shot is. When asking about his childhood, you find that he was born and raised in Colombia. He immigrated to the United States 5 years ago. He does not know if he has ever had a tetanus shot. You inform the physician and he orders diphtheria/tetanus toxoid 0.5 ml IM and Hypertet (tetanus immune globulin) 250 U deep IM.

4. Why is J.O. getting two injections?

5. J.O. has a Foley catheter inserted to drain his urine. What should the nurse assess for in relation to the Foley catheter?

6. While assessing distal to the fractured femur, the nurse notes that his toes are cold to the touch. What other assessment findings should be gathered?

7. J.O. has an antiembolism stockings ordered for his L leg. What is the rationale for putting stockings on only one leg?

8. At 1800 J.O.'s guard summons you to his room. J.O. is cold and clammy, groaning, pale, agitated, and slightly confused. VS are 70/palp, 140, 28, 98.0° F. His pulse is weak and thready. His abdomen is painful and appears to be increased in size. You summon the physician. What else can you do?

9. The physician arrives and wishes to perform a peritoneal lavage. Explain why peritoneal lavage is being done, and describe the procedure.

10. What are the nursing responsibilities in preparation for this procedure (in order)?

11. The physician begins the diagnostic peritoneal lavage procedure. Upon insertion of the trochar into the abdomen, bright red blood under pressure returns. What happens next?

12. In view of the threat made on J.O.'s life and his vulnerable situation, what precautions should the nursing unit take to protect him?

J.O. recovered for several weeks in the hospital before being sent to jail to await trial. Shortly before his trial date, he was found stabbed to death in his cell. Although there was an investigation, the murder weapon was never found, and no one was ever charged in his death.

Case Study 3

Name ______________________ Class/Group ______ Date ______

Group Members ______________________________________

INSTRUCTIONS: All questions apply to this case study. Your responses should be brief and to the point. Adequate space has been provided for answers. When asked to provide several answers, they should be listed in order of priority or significance. Do not assume information that is not provided. Please print or write clearly. If your response is not legible, it will be marked as ? and you will need to rewrite it.

Scenario

You are working on a telemetry unit and have just received a transfer from the ICU. The 50-year-old male patient, T.A., had a repair of an abdominal aortic aneurysm (AAA) measuring 8 cm in diameter. This is his second day postop. He is an attorney with a very active practice. He considered himself to be healthy before diagnosis of the aneurysm, although he took medication for gastritis. He has had progressive weakness of his lower extremities and decreasing urine output since surgery. T.A. also has a 10-year history of type 2 diabetes mellitus (DM); he has been requiring insulin the last 6 months to keep his glucose levels under control.

1. T.A. has questions about his surgery. He asks you, "I was fine before surgery. I'd still be fine now if I hadn't been operated on, wouldn't I?" Based on your knowledge of AAA, what should be your response be?

Because the AAA is clamped during the most crucial part of the surgery, nerve damage to the legs and blood clots are a risk with this surgery and require frequent assessment.

2. You are performing your initial assessment of T.A.'s legs. What findings should you record?

3. Four hours after admission to your floor, you note that T.A. has had a urine output of 75 ml of dark amber urine. You examine the catheter and tubing for obstructions and there are none. What other assessment data should you gather to determine whether or not a problem exists?

4. Laboratory tests reveal renal damage. T.A. is placed on fluid restriction and a renal diet. T.A. asks what he is going to be able to eat on his diet. What is your reply?

5. T.A. has a dialysis catheter inserted into his L subclavian vein. You are preparing to administer an intravenous antibiotic and find that his only other intravenous access, a peripheral line, is obstructed. What should you do?

6. Upon return from his first dialysis, T.A. c/o headache and nausea. He is restless and slightly confused, and he has an elevated BP. You suspect disequilibrium phenomenon. You notify the physician. What nursing measures can you institute at this point?

7. T.A. has an episode of severe vomiting. His abdominal wound dehisces, and a loop of his intestines eviscerates. Another staff member has summoned the doctor. What care should you render before the physician's arrival?

8. You are concerned that the weakness in T.A.'s legs may result in muscle atrophy. What nursing interventions can you take to prevent this?

A sliding scale human recombinant insulin plan has been instituted, but T.A.'s glucose levels have been ranging from 62 to 387 mg/dL. "That's funny," he tells you. "You're giving about the same amount about the same times as I give it to myself at home. I don't understand why it's not working!" You explain to him that the dialysis and the surgery both profoundly affect his insulin needs. In addition, although it may look similar in the syringe, he is getting a different dose of insulin than he has been getting at home.

9. Based on recent findings contrasting the metabolism of human insulin versus animal insulin sources, explain why T.A. may be having trouble regulating his glucose levels.

10. T.A.'s wound is not healing. You call the enterostomal therapy (ET) RN to evaluate what can be done. After looking at T.A.'s wound, he looks at the chart, sighs, and points to the glucose levels. "Here's your problem," he says. "The way this is going, he'll never heal." Based on recent findings in diabetes management, explain what he means. What other health care professionals may help you with T.A.'s glucose regulation?

Case Study 4

Name ________________________ Class/Group ______ Date ______

Group Members ____

INSTRUCTIONS: All questions apply to this case study. Your responses should be brief and to the point. Adequate space has been provided for answers. When asked to provide several answers, they should be listed in order of priority or significance. Do not assume information that is not provided. Please print or write clearly. If your response is not legible, it will be marked as ? and you will need to rewrite it.

❍ ❍ ❍ / ❍ ❍

Scenario

You are working nights on an inpatient geriatric unit. An 82-year-old woman, M.B., is admitted from an extended-care facility with urosepsis, Alzheimer's disease, and a history of hypertension and CVA. Her right side is flaccid. She does not communicate; she moans when in pain; and she hits, kicks, and claws with her left arm and leg when disturbed. Her initial assessment shows emaciation and multiple pressure ulcers. She has an indwelling Foley catheter and one peripheral IV of D_5NS at 75 ml/h. Her initial VS are 86/50, 108, 24, 104.6° F. Her initial WBC is 34.2 cmm.

1. Four hours after admission you note that M.B.'s Foley catheter has not drained any urine. You cannot begin her antibiotics until you collect a urine culture. What should you do? ❍ ❍ ❍ ❍ ❍

2. M.B. has two intravenous antibiotics, gentamicin (Garamycin) and ticarcillin (Ticar), ordered for 1000. Her morning serum creatinine is 3.2 mg/dL. Her admission serum creatinine was 2.0. Which medication can you safely give? ❍ ❍ ❍ ❍ ❍

3. M.B.'s diet is "mechanical soft." The certified nursing assistant (CNA) tells you that M.B. often spits food during feeding. She also becomes agitated and tries to hit and kick the CNA during meals. Her total intake is less than 25% of the food she is supposed to receive. You believe she may be suffering from protein caloric malnutrition. What assessment findings would you gather to support this?

Note: The patient may not be able to handle a mechanical soft diet. You need to consult with an RD to see whether M.B.'s diet needs to be changed to ground or puree.

4. The RD has calculated M.B.'s caloric and protein needs. A PEG tube is inserted, and M.B. is started on continuous tube feedings at 100 ml/h. During your morning assessment you note that her gastric residual is 175 ml. There are no specific orders regarding residual amount. What should you do?

5. M.B. is at high risk for pulmonary aspiration of her tube feedings. What nursing measures can decrease the chances for this complication?

6. M.B. has a large, stage IV decubitus ulcer over her sacrum and stage II decubitus ulcers over both trochanters. You are initiating a turning schedule for M.B. What would be the most effective schedule and position changes?

7. The enterostomal therapy nurse orders an alginate with Tegaderm dressing to the sacral decubitus. What observations are important to note following dressing changes?

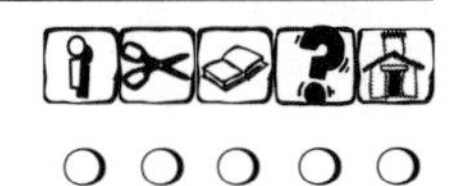

8. What could you do to improve M.B's quality of life? ❍ ❍ ❍ ❍ ❍

Note: So often, basic comfort and pleasure needs of older adults are ignored by our health care system. It is difficult to imagine how miserable life can be when one cannot communicate basic needs and preferences. Unfortunately, you often work with nurses or ancillary personnel who do not have time or interest to investigate these issues.

One of the CNAs at the extended-care facility said M.B. always "perked up" when their therapy dog, Cindy, came for a visit. When Cindy's handler came, she was immediately directed to M.B.'s room. "It was miraculous," the afternoon nurse told her colleague at report, "M.B. perked up and smiled for the first time since she came here. She petted that dog for the longest time and seemed more relaxed and cooperative afterward than you ever could imagine. Maybe all she needed was a little loving. Anyway, they left a picture of Cindy for her to keep on her bedside stand. It seems to have a calming effect on her." Remember, *your* hospital has a therapy dog program too.

Case Study 5

Name ______________________ Class/Group ______ Date ______

Group Members ____

INSTRUCTIONS: All questions apply to this case study. Your responses should be brief and to the point. Adequate space has been provided for answers. When asked to provide several answers, they should be listed in order of priority or significance. Do not assume information that is not provided. Please print or write clearly. If your response is not legible, it will be marked as ? and you will need to rewrite it.

❍ ❍ ❍ / ❍ ❍

Scenario

You are admitting a 30-year-old woman, J.L., to your telemetry unit with the diagnosis of status post-cardiac transplantation and fever of unknown origin (FUO). She was healthy until the birth of her only child at 27 yoa. She developed idiopathic cardiomyopathy following childbirth and underwent cardiac transplantation at 29 yoa. There is a family history of early death from "heart problems."

1. Admitting has assigned J.L. to a semiprivate room. Her roommate is on day 4 of intravenous antibiotic treatment for pneumonia and now has a near normal WBC level. Is this assignment appropriate? What is your response? ❍ ❍ ❍ ❍ ❍

2. Fever is a sign of two major complications of organ transplantation. What are they? ❍ ❍ ❍ ❍ ❍

3. What other s/s of organ rejection should the nurse assess for in this patient? ❍ ❍ ❍ ❍ ❍

4. What other s/s of sepsis should the nurse assess for in J.L.? ❍ ❍ ❍ ❍ ❍

5. While you are assessing J.L., she tells you that she always urinates frequently, because of her diuretics. However, she has experienced burning with urination for the last 2 days. You wish to collect a urine specimen for laboratory analysis. What do you suspect may be causing the burning, and what type of urine specimen should you obtain?

6. The physician tells you that J.L. is to be started on antibiotics as quickly as possible. She has just had a PICC line inserted, and her first dose of intravenous antibiotics has just arrived from the pharmacy. Is there other information that you would like to know before you begin her antibiotics?

7. J.L. says she has complained to her physician that she is constantly SOB running after her 3-year-old. She says her physician told her that this is to be expected but did not tell her why. Why does she become dyspneic with exertion?

8. J.L. tells you that her husband's parents have given her son a pet cat. She jokingly says, "They gave him the play and me the work! My husband is going to have to help. I'm not up to looking after a cat, too." What job does her husband need to do?

9. You would like to teach J.L. some practical things she can do to protect herself from infection. List five. (Hint: this list should include many of the same things cancer patients on chemotherapy are taught.)

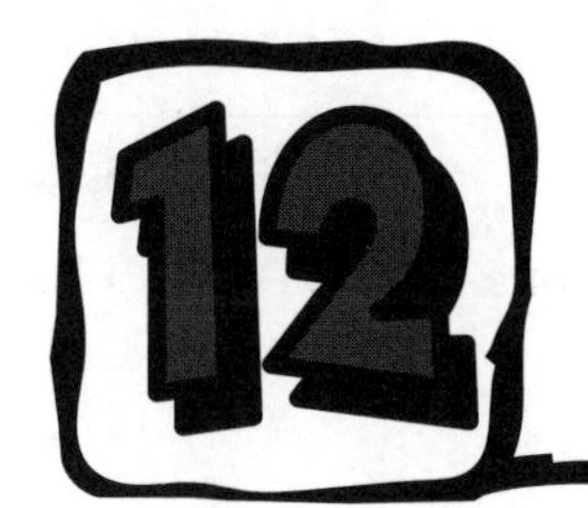

Emergency Situations

Case Study 1

Name ________________________ Class/Group ______ Date ______

Group Members ____

INSTRUCTIONS: All questions apply to this case study. Your responses should be brief and to the point. Adequate space has been provided for answers. When asked to provide several answers, they should be listed in order of priority or significance. Do not assume information that is not provided. Please print or write clearly. If your response is not legible, it will be marked as ? and you will need to rewrite it.

❍ ❍ ❍ / ❍ ❍

Scenario

You are the nurse on a medical unit taking care of a 40-year-old man, T.Z., who has been admitted with peptic ulcer disease (PUD) secondary to chronic alcoholism. You enter T.Z.'s room and find him having a grand mal (tonic-clonic) seizure.

1. List five things you would do. ❍ ❍ ❍ ❍ ❍

Note: Placing any objects, including an airway into the patient's mouth at this point is contraindicated, because of the possibility of patient or caregiver harm.

T.Z.'s seizure activity does not appear to be subsiding, and he is becoming cyanotic. The physician is notified and orders diazepam (Valium) 5 to 10 mg IV until seizure activity subsides.

2. What is the rationale for giving T.Z. diazepam? ❍ ❍ ❍ ❍ ❍

3. What is status epilepticus? ❍ ❍ ❍ ❍ ❍

4. List three things you would be particularly alert for when giving diazepam intravenously.

By the time the physician arrives, T.Z.'s seizure activity has not subsided. The physician administers an additional 10 mg of diazepam, without effect. Fifteen minutes have elapsed since you found T.Z. having seizure activity.

5. What is the significance of this?

The physician decides to administer vecuronium (Norcuron) and intubate T.Z.

6. What is vecuronium, and why is it being administered to T.Z.?

T.Z. has been intubated; the physician orders 600 mg phenobarbital IV and transport to ICU.

7. What is the rationale behind giving phenobarbital?

8. List two nursing problems relataed to T.Z.'s care.

9. Given T.Z.'s history, state at least two possible causes for his grand mal seizure.

T.Z's seizure is successfully treated with diazepam and phenobarbital, and he has no further seizure activity. As you are writing up his release papers, you overhear T.Z. telling his girlfriend to have his car brought to the hospital so he can drive home.

10. How should you respond to this situation? ❍ ❍ ❍ ❍ ❍

Case Study 2

Name ______________________ Class/Group ______ Date ______

Group Members ____

INSTRUCTIONS: All questions apply to this case study. Your responses should be brief and to the point. Adequate space has been provided for answers. When asked to provide several answers, they should be listed in order of priority or significance. Do not assume information that is not provided. Please print or write clearly. If your response is not legible, it will be marked as ? and you will need to rewrite it.

❍ ❍ ❍ / ❍ ❍

Scenario

It is 0800, and the outpatient clinic where you work as an RN has just opened. R.W., a 40-year-old man, hops into the clinic c/o severe pain and swelling in his right lower leg. He tells you he was walking between two cars the night before, when one of the cars was backed up, catching his lower leg between the bumpers. He states he didn't think it was "hurt that bad" and went home to wash the abrasions. He woke up at approximately 0400, and states, "My leg was killing me."

1. How would you transport R.W. to the examining room? ❍ ❍ ❍ ❍ ❍

R.W. is placed in the examining room and asked to remove his trousers and put on a gown. R.W. is unable to lay his leg on the exam table without pain. You observe that his right lower leg is grossly edematous and pale.

2. What should your next priority be? ❍ ❍ ❍ ❍ ❍

There are no pulses in the distal extremity, sensation is diminished, the extremity is cold to touch, and any movement is extremely painful.

3. What should your next action be? ❍ ❍ ❍ ❍ ❍

The physician is with another patient, and asks you to wait a minute.

4. How should you respond? ❍ ❍ ❍ ❍ ❍

After assessing the patient, the physician determines that R.W. should be transported to the nearest ED. The clinic physician notifies the ED physician that R.W. is coming in by ambulance with possible compartment syndrome of the right lower leg.

5. Explain the pathophysiology of compartment syndrome and clarify its significance. ❍ ❍ ❍ ❍ ❍

6. How is compartment syndrome treated? ❍ ❍ ❍ ❍ ❍

7. While waiting for the ambulance, R.W. starts to tell you "one-leg" jokes. How will you respond? ❍ ❍ ❍ ❍ ❍

8. How will you manage the fasciotomy once it has been performed? ❍ ❍ ❍ ❍ ❍

Given that this is a crush injury, the physician orders a urine for myoglobin on R.W.

9. What is the rationale behind this order? ❍ ❍ ❍ ❍ ❍

10. How is rhabdomyolysis treated? ❍ ❍ ❍ ❍ ❍

After an uneventful 5-day stay on the surgical unit, R.W. is being discharged to home care services and has been referred for PT.

11. As you question him about his living conditions, you discover that R.W. lives alone in a third-story apartment; there are no elevators. What other information do you need from him in preparation for discharge?

Case Study 3

Name ______________________ Class/Group ______ Date ______

Group Members ______________________________________

INSTRUCTIONS: All questions apply to this case study. Your responses should be brief and to the point. Adequate space has been provided for answers. When asked to provide several answers, they should be listed in order of priority or significance. Do not assume information that is not provided. Please print or write clearly. If your response is not legible, it will be marked as ? and you will need to rewrite it.

Scenario

You are on duty in the ED when a "code blue" is called overhead. As the code nurse, you grab the crash cart and run to the code, which is in the employee lounge of the operating room. On the couch you find a nurse, Z.H., unconscious, cyanotic, and barely breathing. Her scrub shirt has been cut off, and you attach ECG leads to her chest. Her pulse is 45; respirations are 8 and shallow. She is intubated, an intravenous line is started with 0.9% NaCl, and she is given an ampule of 50 ml D_5W, 0.4 mg naloxone (Narcan), and 0.5 mg atropine IVP. Her respirations improve slightly, and pulse increases to 56. She is transported to the ED.

1. What is the purpose of giving the three drugs mentioned in this case?

After additional naloxone, the patient wakes up and is extubated.

2. What additional information do you want to know?

In response to your questions, Z.H. tells you that she took fentanyl IM. She then asks you to call a friend to come stay with her.

3. What information would you give her friend over the phone?

4. The friend asks you what is wrong. How do you respond?

5. Identify four nursing problems relating to Z.H.'s care that apply to this situation.

Z.H. is admitted to the ICU for 24-hour observation and then transferred to the chemical dependency unit.

6. What is chemical dependency?

One of Z.H.'s colleagues calls on the phone to ask how she is. She tells you that she thought something was wrong with Z.H. because her behavior was so erratic, but "I had no idea it was drugs. I didn't think Z.H. would ever do anything like that!" Keep in mind that patient confidentiality extends to health care professionals not directly involved in Z.H.'s care. You cannot give information on how Z.H. is doing.

7. What is the profile of an impaired nurse? (List five characteristics.)

8. What four problems are associated with impaired nurses who are practicing?

Z.H. asks her nurse what is going to happen to her career.

9. What are the regulatory issues r/t impaired nurses that will guide your response? (List at least five.)

Note: These stipulations vary according to individual state regulatory laws and nurse practice acts. Encourage students to become familiar with the policies of your state.

Z.H. successfully completes treatment and continues to practice as a nurse. She is now serving as a sponsor for another nurse undergoing treatment for chemical dependency.

Case Study 4

Name ____________________ Class/Group ______ Date ______

Group Members ______________________________________

INSTRUCTIONS: All questions apply to this case study. Your responses should be brief and to the point. Adequate space has been provided for answers. When asked to provide several answers, they should be listed in order of priority or significance. Do not assume information that is not provided. Please print or write clearly. If your response is not legible, it will be marked as ? and you will need to rewrite it.

Scenario

J.R. is a 28-year-old man who is doing home repairs. He falls from the top of a 6-foot step ladder, striking his head on a large rock. He experiences momentary loss of consciousness. By the time his neighbor gets to him, he is conscious but bleeding profusely from a laceration over the R temporal area. The neighbor drives him to the ED of your hospital. As the nurse, you immediately apply a cervical collar, lay him on a stretcher, and take J.R. to a treatment room.

1. What steps should you take to assess J.R.?

2. List at least five components of a neuro exam.

You complete your neuro exam and find the following: GCS 15, PERRLA, and full sensation. J.R. c/o a headache; he is becoming increasingly lethargic.

3. As the radiology technician performs a portable cross-table lateral c-spine x-ray, J.R. begins to speak incoherently and appears to drift off to sleep. What is the next action you would take?

You find J.R. has become unresponsive to verbal stimuli and responds to painful stimuli by abnormally flexing his extremities (decorticate movement). He has no verbal response. The right pupil is larger than the left, and does not respond to light.

4. What is J.R.'s GCS score at this time? Indicate what this means.

5. Based on his GCS score, what are the next steps you should take?

6. What is the significance of the dilated and fixed pupil on the right?

The physician orders 500 ml of 25% mannitol solution IV.

7. What is mannitol, and why is it being used on J.R.?

J.R. is transported to CT scan, where he is found to have a large epidural hematoma on the right with a hemispheric shift to the left. He will be taken to the OR from CT scan for evacuation of a right epidural hematoma.

While en route from the CT scan to the OR, the physician instructs the respiratory therapist to initiate hyperventilation of the patient to "blow off more CO_2."

8. What is the rationale for this action?

9. Explain at least six nursing interventions you would use to prevent increased ICP in the first 48 postoperative hours. ❍ ❍ ❍ ❍ ❍

While he is in surgery, J.R.'s family arrives at the ED. They ask that their faith healer anoint J.R. and pray over him.

10. What should the nurse say? ❍ ❍ ❍ ❍ ❍

Case Study 5

Name ______________________ Class/Group ______ Date ______

Group Members ______________________

INSTRUCTIONS: All questions apply to this case study. Your responses should be brief and to the point. Adequate space has been provided for answers. When asked to provide several answers, they should be listed in order of priority or significance. Do not assume information that is not provided. Please print or write clearly. If your response is not legible, it will be marked as ? and you will need to rewrite it.

Scenario

B.J. is a 34-year-old woman who has been thrown from a galloping horse in a remote area. She was flown to the trauma center by helicopter from a rural hospital with spinal cord compression due to spinal fracture and disk fragments in her lumbar spine. Her cervical spine is free from injury. She arrives strapped to a rigid backboard and begins to vomit.

1. What would you do to keep B.J. from aspirating?

Turn her to a side lying position

2. What would you do to assess B.J.?

Take her VS

You find that B.J. is hypotensive and bradycardic. She has an IV of 1000 ml LR with a large-bore catheter at 75 ml/h.

3. What is causing the hypotension and bradycardia?

The neurosurgeon arrives in the ED and examines B.J. He finds her areflexic below the lumbar region of the spinal cord. There is absence of sweating in the region and no sensation below the level of the lesion. He writes the following orders: CT scan of the spine; myelogram; prepare for surgery; admit to ICU; 10 mg dexamethasone (Decadron) IV now.

4. Why did the physician order both a CT scan and a myelogram? Differentiate between the diagnostic value of each.

5. What is dexamethasone, and why is it being used on B.J.?

6. List four nursing problems relevant to B.J.'s care.

7. What are complications and problems associated with spinal cord shock? (List at least six.)

8. List six ways you would detect complications from spinal cord shock.

9. What are seven interventions that could be initiated to prevent or treat complications from spinal cord shock?

B.J. went to surgery directly from x-ray for decompression of her spinal cord, and was admitted to ICU on absolute bed rest. From ICU she was transferred to the surgical unit and fitted for a back brace; she began physiotherapy. After undergoing surgery for a bone graft and spinal fusion, she was transferred to a rehabilitation facility. After months of intense physiotherapy, B.J. regained the use of her legs and basic functioning and was discharged to home.

Case Study 6

Name ______________________ Class/Group ______ Date ______

Group Members ______________________________

INSTRUCTIONS: All questions apply to this case study. Your responses should be brief and to the point. Adequate space has been provided for answers. When asked to provide several answers, they should be listed in order of priority or significance. Do not assume information that is not provided. Please print or write clearly. If your response is not legible, it will be marked as ? and you will need to rewrite it.

❍ ❍ ❍ / ❍ ❍

Scenario

You are working in the ED when a patient comes in with an allergic reaction to bee pollen she has eaten. She brought the jar of bee pollen with her. M.W., your nurse colleague is curious about how bee pollen tastes and ingests a small amount. A few minutes later M.W. begins to experience itching in her throat and ears, hives, and mild respiratory distress. The respiratory distress rapidly progresses to audible wheezing. You notice that she appears to be in distress.

1. What do you think is wrong with M.W.? ❍ ❍ ❍ ❍ ❍

2. Given that your colleague is having a possible allergic reaction, what actions should you take? (List five.) ❍ ❍ ❍ ❍ ❍

3. What is the rationale behind giving the medications you identified in your answer to question 2? List their usual dosages. ❍ ❍ ❍ ❍ ❍

M.W. begins to improve. She states that the itching has subsided and the hives are fading. She reports that she no longer has acute SOB. On auscultation of her lungs, you note that the wheezing has resolved. She wants to return to work.

4. Is it appropriate to allow her to return to duty? Why?

A decision is made to discharge M.W. to her home.

5. What issues should you address in discharge teaching of this nurse? (List three.)

6. Should you allow M.W. to drive herself home? Why?

A friend is called to come and drive M.W. home, and she is discharged. She lives to nurse another day!

Case Study 7

Name ______________________ Class/Group ______ Date ______

Group Members ____

INSTRUCTIONS: All questions apply to this case study. Your responses should be brief and to the point. Adequate space has been provided for answers. When asked to provide several answers, they should be listed in order of priority or significance. Do not assume information that is not provided. Please print or write clearly. If your response is not legible, it will be marked as ? and you will need to rewrite it.

❍ ❍ ❍ / ❍ ❍

Scenario

You are working in an outpatient clinic when a mother brings in her 20-year-old-daughter, C.J., who has type 1 diabetes mellitus (DM) and has just returned from a trip to Mexico. She's had a 3-day fever of undetermined origin (FUO) and diarrhea with N/V. She has been unable to eat and has tolerated only sips of fluid. Because she has been unable to eat, she has not taken her insulin.

Because C.J. is unsteady, you bring her to the examining room in a wheelchair. While assisting her onto the examining table, you note that her skin is very warm and flushed. Her respirations are deep and rapid, and her breath is foul-smelling. C.J. is drowsy and unable to answer your questions. Her mother states "she keeps telling me she's so thirsty, but she can't keep anything down."

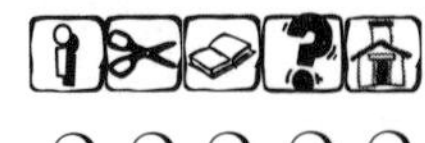

1. List four pieces of additional information you need to elicit from C.J.'s mother. ❍ ❍ ❍ ❍ ❍

2. Describe the pathophysiology of diabetic ketoacidosis. ❍ ❍ ❍ ❍ ❍

3. Explain the patient's presenting s/s (List six.)

4. Her current VS are 90/50, 124, 36 and deep; temperature is 101.3° F (tympanic temp). Are these VS appropriate for a woman of C.J.'s age? Why or why not? Discuss your rationale.

A decision has been made to transport C.J. by ambulance to the local ED. After evaluating C.J., the ED physician writes the following orders.

5. Carefully review each order. Mark with an "A" if the order is appropriate; mark with an "I" if inappropriate. For each order you mark as "I," explain why it is inappropriate and correct the order.

___ 1000 ml LR IV STAT.

___ Give 36 units lente and 20 units regular insulin SC (sub-Q) now.

___ Hemogram with differential; advanced metabolic panel (electrolytes, glucose, enzymes), blood cultures x 2 sites; clean catch urine for UA and C&S; stool for ova and parasites, *C. difficile* toxin, and C&S; serum lactate, ketone, and osmolality; ABGs on room air.

___ 1800-calorie ADA diet.

___ Ambulate qid.

___ Tylenol 650 mg (10 gr) PO.

___ Lasix 60 mg IVP now.

___ Urine output q hour.

___ VS q shift.

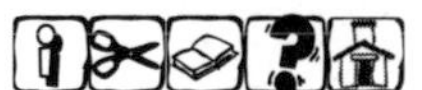

All orders have been corrected and initiated. C.J. has received fluid resuscitation and is on a sliding scale insulin drip via infusion pump. Her latest glucose was 347 mg/dL.

6. What is the rationale behind using an infusion pump for the insulin drip? ❍ ❍ ❍ ❍ ❍

C.J. is ready for transport to the medical ICU. C.J.'s mother is beginning to realize that C.J. is more acutely ill than she thought. She leaves the room and begins to cry.

7. How would you handle this situation? ❍ ❍ ❍ ❍ ❍

8. C.J.'s mother asks where she can get more information on how C.J. can control her diabetes. What are some resources she may find useful? ❍ ❍ ❍ ❍ ❍

C.J. is transported to the MICU in slightly improved condition. She continues to improve and is discharged from the hospital 3 days later.

Case Study 8

Name ________________________ Class/Group ______ Date ______

Group Members ____

INSTRUCTIONS: All questions apply to this case study. Your responses should be brief and to the point. Adequate space has been provided for answers. When asked to provide several answers, they should be listed in order of priority or significance. Do not assume information that is not provided. Please print or write clearly. If your response is not legible, it will be marked as ? and you will need to rewrite it.

Scenario

D.V., a 38-year-old woman diagnosed with ruptured appendix, was hospitalized for an appendectomy. She developed peritonitis and was discharged 9 days later with a left peripherally inserted central catheter (PICC line) to home care for IV antibiotic therapy. You work for the home care department of the hospital. You have been assigned to D.V.'s case, and this is your first home visit. You are to do a full assessment on D.V. During the assessment, you notice a large ecchymotic area over the right upper arm. You question her about the bruise and she tells you, "The nurses took my BP so many times it bruised."

1. Do you accept D.V.'s explanation? Why or why not?

In examining D.V. further, you find a fine, nonraised, dark red rash over her trunk.

2. What questions would you ask D.V. to elicit additional information?

D.V. hadn't noticed the rash before you pointed it out. The rash does not itch or cause pain. She has never had one like it before.

3. What other information would you want to gather?

The wound is not discolored or draining; the abdomen is not tender to deep palpation. There is oozing of serosanguinous fluid around the PICC insertion site. The rash is confined to the trunk. You make a decision to call the physician regarding your assessment findings.

4. What vital information will you relay to the physician? (Always start by identifying yourself.)

The physician orders blood to be drawn for coagulation studies and a CBC with differential. He says he would like to evaluate D.V. for disseminated intravascular coagulation (DIC).

5. What laboratory tests would you expect to see performed in coagulation studies?

You give D.V. her antibiotic, draw her blood, and take it to the lab. You return 6 hours later to administer another dose of antibiotics. D.V. greets you at the door. She is very upset and ushers you to the bathroom, where you find blood in the toilet. She tells you that she has been urinating blood for the past 2 or 3 hours. She also shows you a tissue in which she has bloody-appearing sputum. She tells you she has been coughing up blood. You notify the physician who instructs you to call 911 and get the patient to the ED immediately. You call the ED and give report to the triage nurse on duty.

6. What are you going to tell the triage nurse?

7. Are the patient's presenting s/s consistent with DIC? Explain.

The following labs were prolonged: PT/INR, PTT, split fibrin products, and D dimer. The following labs were decreased: platelets, platelet aggregation time, clot retraction time, and fibrinogen level. CBC is WNR, with the exception of the WBC, which is 12.5 cmm, and platelet count, which is 46 cmm. D.V. is diagnosed with DIC.

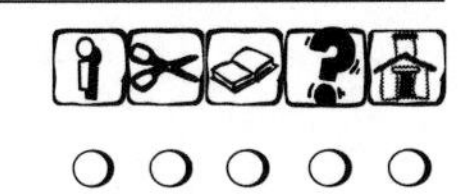

8. List at least three priority needs for D.V.

D.V. is stabilized with oxygen, fluids, and blood products; and medication therapy is initiated. She is transferred to the ICU in guarded condition.

Note: The prognosis for someone with DIC is very poor.

Case Study 9

Name ______________________ Class/Group ______ Date ______

Group Members ______________________________________

INSTRUCTIONS: All questions apply to this case study. Your responses should be brief and to the point. Adequate space has been provided for answers. When asked to provide several answers, they should be listed in order of priority or significance. Do not assume information that is not provided. Please print or write clearly. If your response is not legible, it will be marked as ? and you will need to rewrite it.

Scenario

You are the trauma nurse working in a busy tertiary care facility. You receive a call from the paramedics that they are en route to your facility with the victim of multiple gunshot wounds to the chest and abdomen. The paramedics have started two large-bore IV lines with LR, O_2 by mask at 15 L/minute. The patient has a sucking chest wound on the left and a wound in the upper right quadrant of the abdomen. VS are 80/36, 140, 42. The patient is diaphoretic, very pale, and confused. Estimated time of arrival (ETA) is 4 minutes.

1. List at least six things you will do to prepare for this patient's arrival.

On arrival to the ED, your patient, B.W., is cyanotic and in severe respiratory distress. When he is transferred to the trauma stretcher, you notice that there is an occlusive dressing over the sucking chest wound. It is taped down on all sides.

2. Is taping the occlusive dressing on all sides appropriate? Explain.

3. Who usually responds to a trauma code, and what are the functions of the people from the various departments?

4. Prioritize the actions of the physicians and nurses in the trauma situation.

B.W. is to have a CT scan of the abdomen. His abdomen has become distended and rigid.

5. What are the possible reasons for the abdominal distention and rigidity?

The CT scan shows a large liver laceration. B.W. will be taken directly to the OR for an exploratory laparotomy with repair of liver laceration, then to the ICU. When you return from transporting the patient to the OR, B.W.'s wife is in the ED very upset and frightened. The social worker has been called to another emergency.

6. How would you interact with B.W.'s wife?

Case Study 10

Name ______________________ Class/Group ______ Date ______

Group Members ____

INSTRUCTIONS: All questions apply to this case study. Your responses should be brief and to the point. Adequate space has been provided for answers. When asked to provide several answers, they should be listed in order of priority or significance. Do not assume information that is not provided. Please print or write clearly. If your response is not legible, it will be marked as ? and you will need to rewrite it.

❍ ❍ ❍ / ❍ ❍

Scenario

T.R. is a 22-year-old college senior who lives in the dormitory. His friend finds him wandering aimlessly about the campus appearing pale and sweaty. He engages T.R. in conversation and walks him to the campus medical clinic where you are on duty. It is 1050. He explains to you how he found T.R. and states that T.R. has diabetes and takes insulin. T.R. is not wearing a medical warning tag.

1. What do you think is going on with T.R.? ❍ ❍ ❍ ❍ ❍

2. List two nursing diagnoses for T.R. ❍ ❍ ❍ ❍ ❍

3. What is the first action you would take? ❍ ❍ ❍ ❍ ❍

4. Because the glucometer reading is 50 mg/dL, what would your next action be? ❍ ❍ ❍ ❍ ❍

5. When you enter the room to administer the orange juice, T.R. is unresponsive. What should your next action be?

6. T.R. is breathing at 16 breaths per minute, has a pulse of 85 and regular, but remains unresponsive. What should your next action be if (1) your clinic is well-equipped for emergencies or (2) your clinic has no emergency supplies?

A few minutes after dextrose is administered, T.R. begins to awaken. He becomes alert and asks where he is and what happened to him. You orient him, then explain what has transpired.

7. What questions would you ask to find out what precipitated these events?

T.R. tells you he took 35 units human NPH and 12 units of regular human insulin at 0745. He says he was late to class so he just grabbed an apple on the way. He adds this has happened twice in the past, but he recognized it, treated it with candy, and then ate a meal. He says he is on a 2000-calorie ADA diet (newer research is calling into question the older "ADA calorie diet" approach, but it still is commonly taught and used).

8. Based on your knowledge of different types of insulin, when would you expect T.R. to experience an insulin reaction?

9. List at least four important points that you would stress in discussing your teaching plan with T.R.

Case Study 11

Name ________________________ Class/Group ______ Date ______

Group Members ____

INSTRUCTIONS: All questions apply to this case study. Your responses should be brief and to the point. Adequate space has been provided for answers. When asked to provide several answers, they should be listed in order of priority or significance. Do not assume information that is not provided. Please print or write clearly. If your response is not legible, it will be marked as ? and you will need to rewrite it.

Scenario

You are working on the intermediate cardiac care unit in a large hospital. You are taking care of R.J., who was admitted for a chest contusion he sustained in an auto accident; he fractured the fourth and fifth ribs on his left side. About 2000, his wife runs up to you at the nurse's station and says, "I think my husband just had a heart attack. Come quick!" She follows you into his room, where you find him face down on the floor. He is breathing and is cyanotic from the neck up. His pulse is very weak.

1. What should your first action be?

2. Suddenly, you remember R.J.'s wife, who is anxiously hovering over you in the room. What are you going to do?

The code team arrives. R.J.'s trauma surgeon is making rounds on your unit when the code is called, and he runs to the room. R.J. is intubated, and the NS lock is changed to an IV of LR. The trauma surgeon recognizes Beck's triad and calls for a cardiac needle and syringe. He inserts the needle below the xiphoid process and aspirates 50 ml of unclotted blood.

3. What is Beck's triad, and what causes it?

4. Explain the rationale for the surgeon performing a pericardiocentesis.

R.J. is transferred to the thoracic ICU for observation.

5. As the team prepares R.J.'s transfer, you go to find R.J.'s wife to tell her what has happened. Briefly, and in everyday terms, how would you explain what happend to her husband?

6. As you both get up to leave, Mrs. J. suddenly turns pale and says she feels very dizzy. What are you going to do?

Case Study 12

Name ________________________ Class/Group ______ Date ______

Group Members ____

INSTRUCTIONS: All questions apply to this case study. Your responses should be brief and to the point. Adequate space has been provided for answers. When asked to provide several answers, they should be listed in order of priority or significance. Do not assume information that is not provided. Please print or write clearly. If your response is not legible, it will be marked as ? and you will need to rewrite it.

Scenario

You are the nurse on duty on the intermediate care unit, and you are scheduled to take the next admission. The ED nurse calls to give you the following report, "This is Barb in the ED, and we have a 42-year-old man with lower GI bleeding. He is a sandblaster with a 12-year history of silicosis. He is taking 40 mg of prednisone per day. During the night, he developed severe diarrhea. He was unable to get out of bed fast enough and had a large maroon-colored stool (hematochezia) in the bed. His wife 'freaked' and called the paramedics. He has been seen here and is coming to you. His VS are stable: 110/64, 110, 28, and he's a little agitated. His temperature is 36.8° C. He hasn't had any stools since admission, but his rectal exam was guaiac-positive and he is pale but not diaphoretic. We have him on 5 L O_2/nc. We started a 16-gauge IV with LR at 125/hour. He has an 18-gauge Salem sump to continuous low suction; the drainage is guaiac-negative. We have done a hemogram with differential, advanced metabolic panel, PT/INR and PTT, and a T&C for 4 units RBCs and a UA. He's all ready for you."

1. How should you prepare for this patient's arrival?

K.L. arrives on your unit. As you help him transfer from the ED stretcher to the bed, K.L. becomes very dyspneic and expels 800 ml of maroon stool.

2. What are the first three actions you should take?

K.L. reports that he is getting nauseated but not thirsty. VS are 106/68, 116, 32.

3. What additional interventions would you need to institute?

ABG results are as follows (these results reflect values at sea level): pH 7.45; $PaCO_2$ 33 mmHg; PaO_2 65 mmHg; HCO_3 23 mmol/L; BE +1.0; SaO_2 91%.

4. Interpret the preceding ABGs. What do they tell you?

The gastroenterologist is notified by K.L.'s physician and arrives on the unit to perform a colonoscopy and endoscopy. You are going to give K.L. midazolam (Versed) and meperidine (Demerol) IV during the procedures.

5. Given the above history, what do you think significantly contributed to the GI bleed?

6. What are midazolam and meperidine, and why are they being given to K.L.?

During the colonoscopy, K.L. begins passing large amounts of bright red blood. Hebecomes more pale and diaphoretic and begins to have an altered LOC.

7. Identify five immediate interventions you should initiate.

K.L. has been stabilized with fluids, blood, and FFP. There has been no further evidence of active bleeding. He received ranitidine (Zantac) 150 mg IV push, and is receiving an infusion of 8 mg/h via infusion pump.

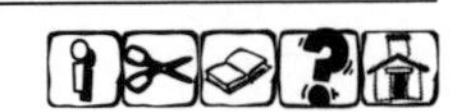

8. Later, when he seems to be feeling better, K.L. tells you he's really embarrassed about the mess he made for you. How are you going to respond to him?

It is concluded that the GI hemorrhage was prednisone-induced. The prednisone is being used to suppress the progression of silicosis. The physician will discharge K.L. and attempt to decrease his maintenance dose of prednisone while monitoring his respiratory status.

Case Study 13

Name ______________________ Class/Group ______ Date ______

Group Members ________________________________

INSTRUCTIONS: All questions apply to this case study. Your responses should be brief and to the point. Adequate space has been provided for answers. When asked to provide several answers, they should be listed in order of priority or significance. Do not assume information that is not provided. Please print or write clearly. If your response is not legible, it will be marked as ? and you will need to rewrite it.

Scenario

S.K., a 51-year-old roofer, was admitted to the hospital 3 days ago after falling 15 feet from a roof. He sustained bilateral fractured wrists and an open fracture of the left tibia and fibula. He was taken to surgery for open reduction and internal fixation (ORIF) of all his fractures. He is recovering on your orthopedic unit. You have instructions to begin getting him out of bed and into the chair today. When you enter the room to get S.K. into the chair, you notice that he is very agitated and dyspneic and says to you, "My chest hurts real bad. I can't breathe."

1. Identify five possible reasons for S.K.'s symptoms.

You auscultate S.K.'s breath sounds. You find that they are diminished in the LLL. S.K. is diaphoretic and tachypneic and has circumoral cyanosis. His apical pulse is irregular and 110 bpm.

2. List in order of priority three actions you should take next.

The physician orders the following: ABGs, chest x-ray (CXR), ECG, and ventilation/perfusion (V/Q) lung scan. The blood gas results come back as follows (these results reflect values at sea level): pH 7.47, $PaCO_2$ 33.6 mmHg, PaO_2 52 mmHg, HCO_3 24.2 mmol/L, BE –3, SaO_2 83%, and A-a gradient 32 mmHg.

3. What is your interpretation of the blood gases? Give your rationale. ❍ ❍ ❍ ❍ ❍

4. Based on the ABGs and your assessment findings, what do you think is wrong with S.K.? ❍ ❍ ❍ ❍ ❍

5. The physician writes the following orders for S.K. Carefully review each order. Mark with an "A" if the order is appropriate; mark with an "I" if the order is inappropriate. Correct all inappropriate orders, and provide rationales for your decisions. ❍ ❍ ❍ ❍ ❍

___ Transfer to MICU.

___ Heparin 20,000 units IVP now, and 20,000 units in 1000 ml/D_5W to run at 1000 units per hour.

___ PT/INR and PTT q4h. Call house officer with results.

___ 3 L O_2/nc.

___ PCA pump with morphine sulfate: loading dose 10 mg; dose 2 mg; lockout time 15 minutes; maximum 4-hour dose 30 mg.

___ Streptokinase 250,000 IU IV over 30 minutes, then 100,000 IU per hour x 48 hours.

___ Solucortef 1 g IV now.

___ Albuterol (Proventil) metered-dose inhaler (MDI), 2 puffs q6h.

All orders have been corrected. S.K.'s V/Q scan indicates a PE in the LLL, and antithrombolytic therapy is initiated. Repeat ABGs show the following values (these results reflect values at sea level): pH 7.45, $PaCO_2$ 35 mmHg, PaO_2 82 mmHg, HCO_3 24 mmol/L, BE –2.4, SaO_2 90%, A-a gradient 28 mmHg.

6. What do these gases generally indicate? ❍ ❍ ❍ ❍ ❍

The physician orders Lasix 20 mg IV now.

7. Why do you think the physician ordered furosemide (Lasix) for S.K.? ❍ ❍ ❍ ❍ ❍

S.K. is watched very closely for the next several days for the onset of pulmonary edema. Thrombolytic therapy, oxygen, pulse oximetry, daily CXRs and ABG analysis, and pain management are continued. When he is stable, S.K. is transferred back to your orthopedic unit.

8. The next day, S.K. suddenly explodes and throws the PT out of his room. He yells, "I'm sick and tired of having everyone tell me what to do." How are you going to deal with this situation? ❍ ❍ ❍ ❍ ❍

Appendix A

Pointers for Students— How to Look Like You Know What You're Doing

Pointers for Students: How to Look Like You Know What You're Doing

Clinical experiences can be overwhelming and confusing; the environment is filled with distractions. What you experience often doesn't resemble what you have read in the book! We want to help you become a good clinician. The following are "tips and tricks" contributed by the writers of these cases. They are presented in no particular order of importance. Don't read all of them at once; read a few here and there, think about them, and apply them as you get the opportunity.

General Suggestions

- There are five instruments every nursing student should carry at all times. Never lend these items to anyone unless you can afford to replace one or more without complaint. These five essential items are a good black-ink ballpoint pen; a high-quality stethoscope; a pocket penlight (preferably with pupil sizes or centimeter ruler on the side); a medium-sized hemostat (straight Kelley); and a pair of bandage scissors.
- Purchase a high-quality stethoscope. Try listening with several different types, and choose the one that is best for you. Engrave your name on it. Your stethoscope is a very important tool.
- Staying hydrated will help you stay more alert. Drink plenty of fluids. (Besides the health benefits, this gives you an excuse to go to the bathroom for 30-second breaks!)
- Keep a quick snack handy. Sometimes you need a pick-me-up and don't have time for meals or to leave the unit to get something.
- Plan something special you can do to help alleviate stress—and use it on a regular basis.
- Avoid use of slang or words that could offend patients and families. Be aware of your patient's comfort level. Do not call patients by their first name unless they have given you permission.
- Assume nothing and take nothing for granted.
- Listen and observe carefully. Be aware of changes and try to anticipate their significance.
- Watch how nurses you work with do things, and pick out things that work best for you.
- You can also learn from a negative example. If nothing else, you learn how *not* to do something!
- Projecting confidence and a "matter of fact" manner will usually put the patient, and yourself, at ease.
- Take care to respect each patient's confidentiality. Conduct interviews and examinations in a private and professional manner.
- Be sensitive to hesitation and nonverbal cues when gathering information. What is left unsaid may be extremely important. Use phrases such as "Could you tell me more?" or "Could you help me understand?" to elicit more information.
- Watch for physical or emotional scars. Health care touches on the most intimate experiences of our lives. Individuals—both men and women—who have been subjected to the degradation of sexual abuse and molestation may be especially prone to shame, aversion, or aggressive reactions.
- Don't be surprised when you discover that many adults are not knowledgeable about the basics of elimination and sexual functioning. Their ignorance or discomfort often is covered up with humor or aggressive behavior.
- Documentation is critical: patient education handouts should be simple to use and developed for use at a sixth-grade reading level.
- If you have a limited budget and a clinical setting of patients who speak more than one language, ask for volunteers to help translate educational material—and then have that work double-checked. Local ethnic clubs or support groups can be a good source of translators.
- As the patient's resting respiratory rate doubles from baseline, he or she will need to be intubated and placed on mechanical ventilation.
- Never trust equipment. Don't assume anything. Things tend to break down at the worst times.
- Double-check to be sure all equipment is functional.
- Treat the patient, not the monitoring devices or numbers.
- Not every patient with hepatitis or cirrhosis is an alcoholic.
- Not every alcoholic will go into DTs.
- Do not assume patients are anorexic just because they look malnourished.
- Do not assume patients are well-nourished just because they are obese.

Assessment and Data Collection

- Learn to assess pain without leaving out important data. Suggestion: use the COLDERRA method where ***C*** = characteristics, ***O*** = onset, ***L*** = location, ***D*** = duration, ***E*** = exacerbation, ***R*** = relief, ***R*** = radiation, and ***A*** = associated signs and symptoms.
- Begin with the basics and keep reviewing them: airway, breathing, circulation (ABCs).
- When you see acute changes in level of consciousness, first check oxygenation status.
- Become a keen observer; use all your senses.
- Don't be distracted by the obvious. Keep looking!

- Formulate a systematic way of assessing patients and make it a habit. Go through the same sequence every time. You will be less likely to overlook or omit something.
- You can't find something if you don't look for it.
- Don't trust (1) machines, (2) numbers, or (3) what you can't see.
- Occasionally ask an experienced nurse or instructor to watch you do your assessments. Everyone, no matter how experienced, can benefit from objective suggestions for improvement. Over time, it is easy to become sloppy or start forgetting important things.
- With the first assessment of your shift, check the patient's ID bracelet and the rate and type of every fluid infusing—you are responsible for fluids under your control from the moment your shift begins until your shift is over.
- Remember to auscultate before palpating: Watch! Listen! *Then* Touch!
- Testing pH of nasogastric tube (NGT) drainage is easier if you slip the litmus paper into the end of the NGT and reconnect the tube to suction. Drainage will be pulled over the paper that can then be removed. (Of course, antacids in the tube will negate this.)
- Any abrupt change in color or amount of drainage from wounds or drains needs to be explored and reported.
- Do not suggest words to describe feelings or events to your patients. You may miss subtle nuances if you jump to conclusions; listen to what your patients have to say and the words they use to say it.
- Perform a thorough psychosocial assessment that includes taking the values of patients and their significant others seriously.
- Include the significant other when you assess sleep patterns. They may be able to tell you more about snoring and other sleep disturbances than the patient can.
- Accurate recording of data, such as intake and output (I&O), is a must. Lawsuits have been won—and lost—over one single I&O sheet. Involve the patient and family in helping to keep accurate records. Ask them to let you know about foods or liquids brought in to the patient.
- Always double-check calculations: use a calculator, if necessary.
- Acute cardiovascular and musculoskeletal injuries require frequent evaluation and documentation of the 5 Ps: Pulse, Pallor, Pain, Paresthesia, and Paralysis. Deterioration of status in any of these variables may indicate a medical emergency and requires a rapid response.
- Be alert for substance abuse as an underlying diagnosis in individuals whose hospitalization is sudden and unanticipated. Many nurses have been injured by patients in undiagnosed withdrawal. This may be a particular risk in motor vehicle accidents (MVAs) or medical crises, where alcohol or drug use may be contributing factors.
- Often, patients and families will deny the existence of mental illness or abuse because of stigma or ignorance. Ask about family violence (verbal or physical) or suicide very carefully.

Understanding the Problem/ Diagnoses

- You have gathered your information, now look at it. Do you see any patterns? Do the data fit the history? Do all medications fit the diagnoses? Are all diagnoses accounted for in the medications?
- Ask the following questions:
  - Do the data make sense in the context of this patient?
  - Do the data create a complete picture?
  - Do you need additional data?
- Use the data to formulate your list of patient problems.
- Prioritize specific problem statements, and guard yourself against distractions.
- Never think you are too smart to look something up.

Developing Strategies of Care

- Plan and coordinate care with your patient. By discussing interventions and priorities, you will learn to understand more about your patient's value system.
- Educate the patient as you carry out this process; process and outcome can and should be integrated. A better educated patient is more prepared to cooperate with the medical and nursing care regimen.
- Always include relationships, cultural orientation, self-esteem, and emotional issues in planning care.
- Prevent infection. Teach your patients and their families to wash their hands properly. Take them to the sink in the room and demonstrate handwashing techniques that you were taught in Nursing 101. Show them how to use a paper towel to turn off the faucet. Have them practice.
- Watch other health care providers to make sure they wash their hands. If you are training others who are with you, leave the water running in the

sink as you leave the room—it is a strong hint for them to wash their hands as they follow you out!

- Check equipment; double-check if you have any doubt. You are responsible for reporting equipment that is not in working order. Equipment not in working order can result in shock or other forms of injury to personnel as well as patients or families. Remove it from the room promptly, label it clearly with a brief description of what is wrong, and report it according to policy.
- Substance abuse is not an uncommon complication in the recovery of trauma patients. Consider a psychiatric nurse practitioner or social services consultation if you suspect this is a problem.
- Accidents or injuries can aggravate feelings and memories associated with earlier experiences of trauma and abuse. If responses to current health problems seem to be unusual or in excess of what is expected, consider consulting a psychiatric nurse practitioner or someone from social services.

Carrying Out the Plan of Care

- Frequently check your patient's charts for STAT orders.
- Document everything you do; if it isn't charted, you didn't do it.
- Document the patient's response to treatments, medications, and activities.
- Let the patient's values and preferences guide you.
- Get the family and significant others to help, if appropriate.

Evaluation and Reevaluation

- Monitor carefully for changes, whether dramatic and sudden, or subtle and gradual.
- Include the patient and families in helping to evaluate care. Ask, "Do you feel that what we are doing is helping you? What do you think?"
- Is the patient getting better? If so, continue with the plan. If not, reassess and revise the plan as needed.
- Evaluate patient and spousal cooperation. Never label patients as "noncompliant." Determine why patients do not take their medication, complete treatments, etc. Perhaps the side effects of treatment make patients feel worse than the disease, and they are exercising their right of choice. Remember, "noncompliance" on the part of patients is more often "knowledge deficit" or ignorance on our part! Noncompliance is rare when there is true teamwork, and it is a misleading term. Adherence is a better, more nonjudgmental word.
- Long-term problems, particularly fatigue and pain, often contribute to depression.
- Involve other health care professionals and pain specialists in addressing complex issues.

Teamwork Is the Key to Survival

- When you graduate and start working as a nurse, you will be expected to be a team leader, coordinating the patient care given by certified nursing assistants, other nurses, and students, with the care given by many other professionals. Use this opportunity to observe the nurses you think are the most effective in promoting teamwork. Analyze why they are effective and try integrating those techniques into your own practice.
- Work at developing good relationships with other professionals. The health care system is complex and constantly changing. We all need and deserve respect. We also depend on one another.
- Getting to know the medical nutritionists (dietitians), pharmacists, physical and occupational therapists, psychologists, social workers, case managers, laboratory personnel, nurse practitioners, medical staff, pastoral counselors, and other professionals in your setting can make things a lot easier for you later on. While you are a student, learn as much as you can about the role of each professional and the most effective ways to interact with them. It all adds up to good patient care.
- Patient care settings can be very stressful, high-pressure environments, especially in emergency situations. Some of the most important things you can remember are:
  - Try to sort out the difference between fact and feelings.
  - Be forgiving.
  - Never take anything personally.

Appendix B

Case Study Worksheet—Preparation and Self-Correction

Case Study Worksheet: ___ Preparation ___ Self-Correction

Name: ________________________________ Chapter _____ Case _____ Date _____________

Patient initials _______

Symbols/terms/abbreviations	Meaning/definition (diagnoses and medications go in following sections)

Diagnoses/medical conditions (+current and –past)	Description/meaning of diagnosis or medical problem (include possible significance)

Medications (brand and generic name if applicable)	Class, indications, contraindications, significant side effects, food and drug interactions

Treatments, interventions and therapeutic procedures	Method of delivery, purpose/desired outcome, indications, contraindications, and precautions (include supplemental oxygen, tube feedings, therapeutic beds, etc.)

Laboratory tests and diagnostic procedures	What is it, when was it done, and why?

Cultural issues and their significance:

Notes:

Appendix C

Self-Correction—Process Worksheet

Self-Correction—Process Worksheet

Name: ______________________________ Chapter _____ Case _____ Date ____________

Questions revised on this workSheet: ___, ___, ___, ___, ___

Question # ___

Revision: ____

○ ○ ○ ○ ○

Question # ___

Revision: ____

○ ○ ○ ○ ○

Question # ___

Revision: ____

○ ○ ○ ○ ○

Question # ___

Revision: ______________________________

Question # ___

Revision: ______________________________

Overall evaluation: ❍ ❍ ❍ / ❍ ❍

Additional feedback from instructor: ______________________________

Permission for unrestricted number of copies of this form may be made for use in conjunction with this book and corresponding clinical use by legitimate owners of this book only.